GANDHI

THE VEGETARIAN

GANDHI'S MESSAGE OF
NON-VIOLENCE,
NON-ABUNDANCE,
AND MERCIFUL LIVING

Holly Hadlayne Roberts

Gandhi

The Vegetarian

Gandhi's message of non-violence, non-abundance, and merciful living

Written and Illustrated by
Holly Harlayne Roberts, D.O., PhD

Anjeli Press

GANDHI

THE VEGETARIAN

GANDHI'S MESSAGE OF NON-VIOLENCE, NON-ABUNDANCE, AND MERCIFUL LIVING

Written and Illustrated
by Holly Harlayne Roberts, D.O., Ph.D.

Published by Anjeli Press
www.Anjelipress.com

ISBN 0-9754844-9-4

Printed in the United States of America
by Lightning Source
Distributed by Ingram Distributors

Written in the hope that,

someday,

Humankind will recognize

the Wisdom of

Non-Violence,

Non-Abundance,

and Mercifully Living.

ACKNOWLEDGEMENTS

Mahatma Gandhi

Mohandas K. Gandhi, 1869–1948, also known as Mahatma Gandhi, the Great Soul, or Gandhiji, the Honorable Gandhi.

The man who led India to independence in 1947 through nonviolent means. A man of strong faith, an individual with unwavering belief in nonviolence, and a vegetarian.

The Government of India

For collecting the speeches given, and the articles and letters written, by Mahatma Gandhi into the one hundred volume compendium, *The Collected Works of Mahatma Gandhi*. It is because of this effort that the world has been better able to understand and learn from this great man.

TABLE OF CONTENTS

Introduction XI

PART ONE
THE PLANTING OF SEEDS

Chapter 1 ... Gandhi's Youth 1
Chapter 2 ... Gandhi's Hindu Faith............................ 7
        Principles of Hinduism................................... 10
        God in All Beings....................................... 15
        Laws of Karma and Rebirth 17
Chapter 3 ... Principles Gandhi valued from Other Faiths ... 21
        The Jain Faith 23
        The Buddhist Faith 25
        The Christian Faith....................................... 27

PART TWO
THE CULTIVATION OF VALUES

Chapter 4... Gandhi's Belief that God Exists in All Beings .. 31
Chapter 5... Gandhi's Philosophy of Non-Violence 35
Chapter 6... Gandhi's Philosophy of Non-Abundance 43

PART THREE
THE SPROUTING OF BELIEFS

Chapter 7... Gandhi's Philosophy of a Healthly Lifestyle..... 49
Chapter 8... Gandhi's Philosophy of a Healthy Diet 54
        Categories of Diets 58
        Grains 59
        Cereals 60
        Rice.. 61
        Pulses: Peas and Beans................................ 62

Vegetables... 64
Fruit 68
Fats: Oil, Butter, Ghee................................ 70
Milk 72
Eggs 77
Sugar... 79
Condiments.. 80
Tea, Coffee, Cocoa 81
Alcohol 83
Animal Flesh 84
Frequency of Meals...................................... 89
Quantity of Food 90
Self-Restraint.. 93
Fasting 95
Tolerance for Non-Vegetarians.................... 97

PART FOUR
SUMMARY & CONCLUSION

Chapter   9 ... Mahatma Gandhi: The Vegetarian................ 101
                Gandhi's Message of Non-Violence,
                Non-Abundance & Merciful Living
Chapter 10 ... Mahatma Gandhi: The "Great Soul" 105

BACK MATTER

End Notes 113
Glossary of Terms 121
References 125

INTRODUCTION

Gandhi was a humble man. He was not the sort of man one would have thought would bring freedom to his country, would alleviate the plight of the untouchables, or would show the world a means by which to deal with conflict without resorting to violence. But he was.

As a youth, he did not shine in school. He disappointed his father, and then lost him at a young age. When sent to college to become a physician, he failed in every class. He graduated law school, but then failed as a lawyer. He was thrown off a train in Africa because of his skin color. He lived his life working for social causes without pay. And he died penniless.

You may ask, "So who was Gandhi?" "Was he a saint?" "No, not at all." "Did he claim to be perfect?" "No, he certainly did not." "Was he always right?" "No, not that either." You see, he was just a man. An honest, quiet, frail, questioning, and humble man.

He was just a man who tried to understand what was right. And do it! He tried to be fair, non-judgmental, non-violent, truthful, and kind. He was a selfless man. He tried to free his people, yet not hurt their enemies. He tried to spare the lives of weaker beings, yet not affect the welfare of humans. He tried to help the intouchables, the suffering masses of humanity in his own country, yet not blame those who had made them suffer. He tried to help others see that all humanity must strive to help one another, or all will succumb. And he succeeded, only partially.

And it is because Gandhi succeeded only partially that his message needs to live on. It needs to be continually retold to all humanity so that its seeds of wisdom might spread and disseminate far and wide, and bud into lofty concepts. Then hopefully, someday, humankind will humble itself to the earth, and no longer abuse its fellow human beings, its brethren animal beings, and its planet.

Was Gandhi a Vegetarian? Yes, of course he was. Why wouldn't he be? He was born into a vegetarian family, lived in a vegetarian country, and belonged to a vegetarian faith. He, himself, acknowledges that this was the initial reason he had been vegetarian. But as his values began to mature, he became a vegetarian by choice. By a strong choice!

When still a child at home, Gandhi never even saw animal flesh. Then, as a young man with friends, he first attempted to eat meat. He actually tried several times. The main reason, however, that he just could not continue was simple. He felt guilty! He knew the pain his parents would suffer if they found out.

Then, at nineteen years of age as a student in England, Gandhi began to question the reasoning behind his vegetarianism. Having suddenly been placed in a nation of non-vegetarians, he was forced to look within and question his own values.

He began to delve into the wisdom of the ancient Hindu faith into which he had been born and formulate his own values based upon this. Over time, he recognized that his faith taught him to perceive the essence of God within each being, and to value the concepts of non-violence, non-abundance, and truth. To Mahatma Gandhi, being vegetarian was not a matter of health or longevity, it was a matter of principle.

[It was] for the building of the spirit and not of the body.

Gandhi, *Harijan*, 20 February 1919[1]

Gandhi was born, lived, and died, a humble man. He did not consider his achievements great, or even consider them his own. Rather, he considered them the will of God.

We achieve only as much as it is our good fortune to do. Our only right is to determined effort.

Gandhi, *The Bhagavad Gita*[2]

Through this look into Gandhi's philosophy of life, truth, non-violence, non-abundance, and vegetarianism, one will gain insight into the hopes and dreams that this humble, sincere man shared for the people of India, for humankind, for all creatures, and for all creation.

Service to all living beings may be said to be the object of human life.

Gandhi,
Letter to Avadhesh Dutt Avasthi
24 May 1935[3]

PART ONE

THE PLANTING

OF SEEDS

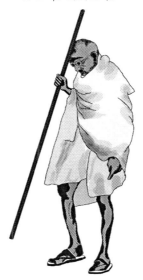

The only basis for having a vegetarian society and proclaiming a vegetarian principle is, and must be, a moral one.

Gandhi, *Harijan*, 20 February 1919 [1]

PART ONE

THE PLANTING OF SEEDS

CHAPTER 1: GANDHI'S YOUTH

Mohandas Karamchand Gandhi was born in 1869 in the State of Gujarat, in Western India. On reflecting back to his youth, he recalls that from the time he was six or seven years of age, until he was sixteen, he learned everything in school, except religion. He felt that the religious values he did acquire were those he passively absorbed during his very early years at home.

Gandhi remembers his mother as a deeply religious woman. The impression she left on him was one of saintliness. She would not take her meals without saying prayers, went to temple regularly, observed religious holidays, and fasted often.[2]

Gandhi's father had been married three times. His wives from his first two marriages passed on while quite young. His final marriage was to Gandhi's mother. Gandhi described his father as a man of truth, courage, and generosity, who never harbored a desire for power or wealth. As a result, he left the family with many high level values, yet very little property. Although Gandhi's father had little academic or religious education, he possessed a strongly religious mind set, and brought the family to Hindu temples and religious discourses frequently. It was not until his last days, however, that Gandhi's father began to read the *Bhagavad Gita*.

Gandhi's father taught him the meaning of unconditional love and compassion. Gandhi recalls one such example from his youth. It was during a time when he had become involved with a classmate of questionable values. Along with this classmate, Gandhi stole money from his family's servants to purchase meat. Entrapped in his own guilt, he wanted to tell his father, yet feared the pain it would cause him. Instead, Gandhi wrote a letter of confession to him. In it, he asked for punishment, and then for forgiveness.

Gandhi silently handed the slip of paper to his father. His father had been ill at the time and was confined to bed. When his father read it, pearl-drops of tears trickled down his cheeks wetting the paper. His father then closed his eyes, lay back down, and tore up the paper. Gandhi felt that those tears were pearl-drops of love. They cleansed his heart and left an indelible impression of love, kindness, and *ahimsa* on his soul.[3]

Having been born in the *Vaishnava* branch of the Hindu faith, Gandhi was taken to the *Haveli* (*Vaishnava*) Temple often. Although he went to temple, the glitter and pageantry of it never appealed to him. He felt disillusioned with religion because of this. As a result, for a good deal of his youth, he lost interest in religion.[4]

As a child, Gandhi suffered from shyness and hesitancy in speech. Initially, he considered these a weakness. Over time, however, he recognized that this affliction had taught him economy of words. It fostered in him the habit of restraining his words, and spared him from overstepping his bounds in speech. Because of this, he grew to recognize silence as a spiritual discipline of truth.

Gandhi observed that when speaking, it is a natural weakness of man to exaggerate, to suppress, or to modify truth. Silence enables one to surmount this weakness. He believed that most of the time, talking was of little benefit to the world, and concluded that his shyness allowed him to grow in his discernment of truth.[5]

Gandhi felt that the seeds that were to eventually grow into his philosophy of vegetarianism had been sown during his early childhood. Although he had been innately oriented towards idealism, Gandhi was inspired through his readings of spiritually inspired texts and by the guidance given him by his family and friends.[6]

When he was still a youth, a wave of reform began to sweep India. The masses thought that if the entire country took to meat-eating, they would become strong and daring enough to overcome the British. This turn away from vegetarianism had nothing to do with pleasing the palate. Rather, it was considered a matter of duty. Gandhi, too, believed it to be a matter of duty. Yet he also felt there was a more significant principle of trust in this act, for he did not want to betray his parent's trust. Nevertheless, Gandhi went to a lonely spot by a river, and there, saw meat!

It was goat's meat. Gandhi tried to eat, but found it as tough as leather. He felt terrible. Even the thought of eating it made him sick. He had to stop. He was haunted by terrible nightmares that entire night of a goat bleating inside him. During the following year, he was coaxed several more times into thinking it was his duty to eat meat. Finally, he could not bear it any longer. Knowing how sad his parents would be if they knew he had eaten meat, he said to himself:

Though it is essential to eat meat, and also essential to take up food 'reform' in the country, yet deceiving and lying to one's father and mother is worse than not eating meat. In their lifetime, therefore, meat-eating must be out of the question.

Gandhi, *Key to Health* [7]

At the age of thirteen, Gandhi was married to his cousin, Kasturbai. Though not fully prepared for such a commitment, he harbored a lifelong sense of faithfulness towards her. She remained his wife and trusted companion for life.

In describing his youth in Gujarat, India, Gandhi explained that his family possessed a strong commitment to vegetarian non-violence. Many of the family's beliefs concerning non-violence were similar to those of followers of the Jain faith. The Jain faith was strong in Gujarat, where Gandhi grew up. He felt its influence everywhere and at all times.

Gandhi believed that because of the combined values of those of the Jain and the *Vaishnava* Hindu faiths, the opposition to and repulsion against eating meat was stronger in Gujarat than in any other region of the world, either inside or outside of India. Followers of both faiths possessed strong commitments concerning the sanctity of all life. These were the traditions in which Gandhi was born and bred. [8]

Hindus are again divided into four chief castes, viz., the Brahmins, the Kshatriyas, the Vaisyas, and the Sudras. Of all these, only the Brahmins, and the Vaisyas are pure vegetarians.

Gandhi, T*he Vegetarian*, 7 February 1891 [9]

Once when Gandhi was traveling in India, his friend brought him to a Kali temple. There, he saw a flock of sheep being brought to slaughter. When he approached the temple, a stream of blood greeted him. He felt so repulsed that he could not bear to stand there. He never forgot the sight.

He asked the others, "Do you regard this sacrifice as religion?" It was then that Gandhi resolved that the more helpless the creature, the more it was entitled to protection by men, rather than to cruelty by men.[10]

When Gandhi reached sixteen years of age, a cloud seemed to shroud his life. First, his father passed away. Shortly after that, his wife and he had a baby that lived only a few days and then died. He searched for meaning. He found this in his spiritual-philosophical belief that, "There is orderliness in the Universe, there is an unalterable Law governing everything and every being that exists or lives." [11] He described this Law as God or Truth.

> *I do dimly perceive that whilst everything around me is ever changing, ever dying, there is underlying all that change a living Power that is changeless, that holds all together, that creates, dissolves, and recreates. That informing Power or Spirit is God. And since nothing else I see merely through my senses can or will persist, He alone is. Hence I gather that God is Life, Truth, Light. He is Love. He is the supreme Good.*
>
> Gandhi, "*God Is*" *Young India*,
> 11 October 1928 [12]

SITE WHERE GANDHI WAS BORN AND RAISED

GUJARAT, INDIA

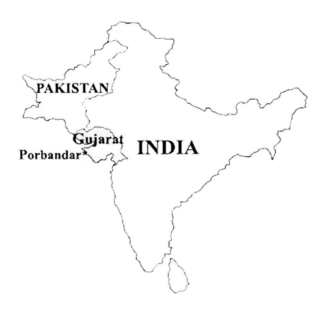

Gandhi's family was from Porbandar in the State of Gujarat, on the west coast of India.

CHAPTER 2: GANDHI'S HINDU FAITH

At nineteen years of age, Gandhi was sent to England to study law. There, he began to learn about Western values, customs, and religion. While studying other faiths, he came to the realization that he had never really learned his own.

He decided to make a dispassionate study of all religions, and before embracing any other faith, he should fully understand his own.[13] This was the first time he ever read the *Bhagavad Gita*, the sacred Hindu text that became his Bible.[14]

> *Believing as I do in the influence of heredity, being born in a Hindu family, I have remained a Hindu.*
>
> *I should reject it if I found it inconsistent with my spiritual growth. On examination I have found it the most tolerant of all religions known to me.*
> Gandhi, *Young India*, 20 October 1927 [15]

Through his studies of the Hindu sacred texts, specifically the *Bhagavad Gita,* Gandhi formulated his own personal philosophy of life. This philosophy would remain with him throughout his life. It led him on his life-long quest seeking peace at every level of existence through the practice of non-violence, non-abundance, and merciful living. Thus he began his mission—a mission that would change our world.

In explaining why he valued Hinduism, the faith he was born into, Gandhi said he found it the most inclusive and all-embracing of all religions. Hinduism is not an exclusive religion. It teaches that God is so great and so miraculous that God can manifest in an infinite number of ways to all different people, and does!

This philosophy enables Hindus to respect other religions, and to embrace the values of other faiths as one of a multitude of variations of paths to the realization of God.

Gandhi also felt that although the concept of non-violence is common to all religions, it found its highest expression in Hinduism.

> *The qualities which you attribute to me are not certainly the result of this* [formal] *education. I am what I am, by the study of my religion and eternal principles of life and such religious and philosophical books as the Bhagavad Gita, Mahabharata, and Ramayana.*
>
> Gandhi, *Discourses on the Gita*,
> 4 July 1926 [16]

To Gandhi, "the Hinduism" that was dear to him was simple, pure Hinduism. It was free of the misguided layers of interpretations that humankind had added to it over the millennia.

> *I am a Hindu by birth and I find peace in the Hindu religion.*
>
> Gandhi, *Discourses on the Gita*,
> 24 December 1926 [17]

To Gandhi, Hinduism was a religion of truth, non-violence, and mercy. He also noted that the greatest Hindu reformers were men of non-violence and were, invariably, vegetarians.

> *The greatest Hindu reformers have been the activist in their generation and they have invariably been vegetarian.*
> Gandhi, *Young India*, 7 October 1926 [18]

He felt that the foundational values of Hinduism that had survived over five thousand years were the truths of the Hindu faith. [19]

> *Hinduism and my conception of the Gita, of the Vedas, the Upanishads, the Bhagavata, and the Mahabharata, teach me that all life is one, and that in the eye of God there is no superior and no inferior.*
> Gandhi, *The Hindu*, 28 January 1933 [20]

Gandhi believed that one of the "truths" of Hinduism, and, therefore, one of its gifts to the world, was vegetarianism.

> *Vegetarianism is one of the priceless gifts of Hinduism.*
> Gandhi, Young India, 7 October 1926 [21]

PRINCIPLES OF HINDUISM

To understand the moral, ethical, and spiritual values that initially inspired Gandhi to embark upon his lifelong path of non-violence towards all beings, and hence, to vegetarianism, one would do well to gain a foundational understanding of the Hindu faith.

Hinduism is a highly-evolved and deeply philosophical religious faith. It is the most ancient of all the major religions of the world, having originated over 7,000 years ago.

In Hindu philosophical thought, all aspects of creation are integrally related to all others within the cyclic, infinite continuum of time and space. All creation exists amidst a continuous flow of recycling birth, life, death, and rebirth. New beings could not exist were it not for their passing on in prior lives. The future could not exist, were it not for the departing of the past.

Based upon such beliefs, Gandhi recognized that all creation is of one essence.

> *The chief value of Hinduism lies in holding to the actual belief that All life is one, i.e. All life comes from the One Universal Source. The unity of All life is a peculiarity of Hinduism which confines salvation not to human beings alone but says that it is possible for all God's creatures. It may be that it is not possible, save through the human form, but that does not make man the Lord of creation. It makes him the servant of God's creation.*
> Gandhi, *Harijan*, 26 December 1936 [22]

Within this cyclic flow of creation, the soul of each being is merely a tiny speck within the unified, infinite continuum of creation. Based upon such beliefs, Gandhi considered all beings to be his brothers:

> *Universal brotherhood—not only brotherhood of all human beings, but of all living beings.*
>
> Gandhi, Kottayam Speech, *Harijan*,
> 30 January 1937 [23]

In Hinduism, a portion of the soul of God exists within each and every being. Each soul feels joy, pain, peace, and fear, just as does every other soul. Each soul possesses the same needs and sensitivities as does every other soul, for all are of the same essence. When one soul suffers, all souls suffer. All emanate from God.

> *I hope every one of you realizes the seriousness and magnitude of the mission that I am trying to carry out in the name of God. . . . There can be, in God's eyes, no distinction between man and man even as there is no distinction between animal and animal.*
>
> Gandhi, Speech at Public Meeting, Madras
> *The Hindu*, 21 December 1933 [24]

In the end, just as all souls emanate from God, all souls will, someday, return to God. All are of the same essence.

> *I want to identify myself with everything that lives.*
>
> Gandhi, My Mission, *Young India*,
> 3 April 1924 [25]

Background of the Hindu Faith

The wisdom of Hinduism began and evolved amongst the holy sages living within the far reaches of the Himalayan mountain range of Northern India. Legend has it that this wisdom was brought down from the mountains by Uma, the wise and beautiful daughter of one of these sages.

Looking beyond the legend, the fact remains that the ancient wisdom of Hinduism, that is the wisdom of the Hindu *Vedas*, evolved amongst the spiritually advanced sages native to the mountains of northern India. These people had lived for centuries in what is considered present-day Punjab. Over centuries, the wisdom of the *Vedas* was disseminated amongst the people living along the banks of the Sindhu (Indus) River and Saraswati River in northwest India. [26]

The highly-evolved civilization of the mountain sages, later known as the "Aryan Civilization," and the civilization of those living along the river banks, later known as the "Indus Valley Civilization," were populated by people native to the Indian sub-continent.

The *Vedas* teach that God created all, God is in all, and God is all! God is within every person, every animal, and every aspect of creation.

> *All that there is in this Universe, great or small,*
> *including the tiniest atom, is pervaded by God,*
> *known as creator or Lord.*
> Gandhi, *Harijan*, 30 January 1937 [27]

Over the centuries, Hinduism's sacred scriptures grew to encompass three basic works: The *Vedas*, the *Puranas*, and the epics.

The *Vedas* are the foundational, sacred teachings of Hinduism. Within these, the *Upanishads* are the final portion of each. They contain the philosophical wisdom of the *Vedas*.

The *Puranas* are a voluminous collection of Hindu mythology filled with spiritual and moral lessons.

The Epics, the *Ramayana, Mahabharata,* and *Bhagavad Gita*, are epic tales that express the philosophical, moral, and spiritual teachings of the Hindu faith.

Gandhi admitted that he never made an in depth study of all the *Upanishads*, but benefited greatly from those he had. He read the *Isha Upanishad* while imprisoned in Yeravda Jail and learned it by heart.[28]

He believed that if all the other *Upanishads* were somehow lost, the *Isha Upanishad* would sustain the Hindu faith. It conveys the message that one's life should be a life of continual service to one's fellow beings.[29]

The *Isha Upanishad* also tells that although humans may think they are special, and other beings lowly, all are physically and spiritually one.

The ant and the elephant, the Brahmin and the sweeper, man and woman, the bodies of them all are composed of clay and other things. The Upanishads and other scriptures teach us that an inward view will reveal only one soul pervading us all.

Gandhi, *Hindi Navajivan*, 31 October 1929 [30]

It was the *Bhagavad Gita*, however, that Gandhi considered his spiritual guide.

The *Bhagavad Gita* teaches that all life is unified in a cyclic continuum with all that has ever lived, presently lives, and will ever live. Valuing this philosophy, Gandhi considered it his duty not to kill or harm any being. He felt a kinship with all.

My ethics do not permit me to claim but require me to own kinship with not merely the ape, but the horse and the sheep, the lion and the leopard, the snake and the scorpion.

Gandhi, More Animal than Human,
Young India, 8 July 1926 [31]

PRINCIPLES OF HINDUISM

GOD IN ALL BEINGS

Of the foundational concepts within Hinduism that guided Gandhi along his life journey of non-violence toward all people and all beings was its teaching that God is present in all beings.

Within the Hindu faith, God is envisioned as being present within every person, every being, and every thing. God is so all encompassing that God is present within all that is above and all that is below, within all that moves and all that is still, within all that is seen and all that is unseen. God is embodied within all that lives, breathes, and feels. And because God is present within all creation, each and every aspect of creation is of value. Each embodies the soul of God.

> *All embodied life is in reality an incarnation of God.*
>
> Gandhi, *The Bhagavad Gita* [32]

The Hindu faith evolved as a faith over thousands of years. And so, too, did the Hindu concept of God. In Hinduism, God is not away and apart from all that God created, God is present in all. God is in the tiniest grain of sand and in the widest expanse of sky. God is also in the hearts of all.[33] It is God, amidst the multitude of all that God has created, that a Hindu worships. A Hindu respects all beings, as each contains the essence of God.

Every object and every state which we can think
of in this universe are God.
                    Gandhi, *The Bhagavad Gita* [34]

Based upon the realization that God is in all, Hindus consider it the highest virtue to be nonviolent toward all beings and all creation. One of Hindu faith cannot envision harming or taking the life of any being.

There can be no two opinions on the fact that
Hinduism regards killing a living being as sinful.
          Gandhi, *Young India*, 21 October 1926 [35]

Archeological and astronomic events narrated in the *Vedas*, such as volcanic and seismic upheavals, and the patterns of stars, definitively reveal that the *Vedas* were composed, at least in oral form, prior to 5,000 BCE. The *Upanishad*s are the philosophical portion of each *Veda*.

The *Upanishads* are considered the teachings of God transmitted to humankind through Rishis, or ancient seers of truth.[36] These teachings are considered truths that have existed since the beginning of time.[37]

The *Upanishads* explain Hinduism's concepts of God, *karma*, rebirth, nonviolence, and the soul. They teach that the Soul of God pervades the entire universe, and also exists within the soul of each and every being. God is present in all things, those seen and those unseen. God is the past, the present, and the future. God is all that can be conceived, imagined, or dreamed. All creation is, in essence, the Soul of God. [38]

PRINCIPLES OF HINDUISM

LAWS OF KARMA AND REBIRTH

The *Law of Karma* and the *Law of Rebirth* are fundamental principles within Hinduism. They are much deeper concepts than the Western concept of, "As a man sows, so shall he reap."

In addition, they are inextricably intertwined with one another. To understand both of these concepts, one must initially understand the Hindu concept of the soul.

In Hindu philosophy, a soul exists within each being. Each soul emanates from, and is part of, the Universal Soul of God. This Soul has always permeated all existence.

The Universal Soul pervades all that exists, all that has ever existed, and all that will ever exist. It is eternal and immortal. The soul within each being emanates from the Universal Soul, and because of this, the soul within each individual is eternal and immortal as well.

The *Law of Rebirth* teaches that each soul is reborn again and again into a series of lives. The challenges that each soul must face have been determined by its thoughts, words, and actions in that soul's many prior lives.

> *For I believe in rebirth as much as I believe in the existence of my present body. I therefore know that even a little effort is not wasted.*
> Gandhi, *Young India*, 5 June 1924 [39]

Similarly, the actions each soul performs during its present life will affect the fate that soul encounters in all its future lives.[40]

One's actions are termed '*karma*.' The Hindu term '*karma*' refers both to one's actions and to the results of one's actions. The *Law of Karma* places the responsibility for one's actions (one's *karma*) directly upon oneself. From a karmic perspective, one's 'actions' include all of one's thoughts, words, and deeds.

> *Every thought is a form of Karma.*
> Gandhi, *Bhagavad Gita* [41]

As one thinks, so will one act, and so will one become. One's actions will affect the fate of one's soul in one's present life, and in all of the future lives that one's soul may experience—infinitely until that specific soul is purified. One's actions, indirectly, also affect the fate of all the other souls with which one's soul comes in contact.

Recognizing the karmic effects that will occur due to one's actions, now and throughout infinity, one is humbly guided towards a life of compassion and nonviolence towards all people, all beings, and all creation.

According to the Hindu *Law of Karma*, all that occurs throughout eternity does so as a result of both the personal and the collective *karma* of all. Though one cannot normally recall what has occurred within one's soul's prior existences, God remembers all!

One should ensure that all of one's thoughts, words, and deeds are pure, kind, and meaningful in content, for

> *Karma can never be undone. All actions bear fruit, good or bad.*
>> Gandhi, Letter to Devdas Gandhi,
>> 24 July 1918 [42]

So too, did Gandhi recognize that all life was of one karmic interrelated breath. He believed that the suffering one might inflict upon a weaker creature would not only harm that weaker being, but would also impart a karmic blot on one's own soul. It would also impart a karmic blot upon all creation, during the present time and during all future times. [43]

In addition, the *Laws of Karma* and *Rebirth* teach that if one commits a dishonest or cruel action, one's soul must return for another lifetime to repent for and repay for that misdeed. The characters involved in the subsequent lifetime may externally appear different, and one may not know that one is repaying a karmic debt, but there is no doubt—a karmic debt will be repaid.

> *All creation appears and vanishes, and does so endlessly. The round of birth and death is ceaseless.*
>> Gandhi, *The Bhagavad Gita* [44]

Recognizing this, Gandhi felt sympathy with all beings facing challenges, whether that being was human or non-human.

> *We should not serve anyone with the hope that he, too, will serve us one day, but we may serve him because the Lord dwells in him. If we hear anyone crying in distress for help, we should immediately run to him and help him. We should help the Lord crying in distress.*
>
> Gandhi, *Bhagavad Gita* [45]

As a Hindu, Gandhi recognized that the soul of each being was bound within its own eternal continuum, yet each soul was also bound to the Universal Soul.[46]

> [We must] *learn to identify ourselves with all that lives. The sum total of that lives is God. Hence, the necessity of realizing God living within every one of us.*
>
> Gandhi, *The Diary of Mahadev Desai*, 21 June 1932 [47]

CHAPTER 3

PRINCIPLES GANDHI VALUED FROM OTHER FAITHS

Gandhi was a devoutly religious Hindu. Nevertheless, he valued the spiritual and moral wisdom of all other faiths. He read, studied, and absorbed the teachings of non-violence of the Jain, Buddhist and Christian faiths. He then incorporated many of these into his personal philosophy.

He preferred not to compare the merits of different faiths. Rather, he spent his time reading the holy books of each faith, and then praying.[48] His father taught him tolerance for all branches of Hinduism, and for all other faiths. His parents would visit Haveli, Shiva, and Rama temples, and frequently invite Jain monks to visit their home. They had friends of many faiths, and would discuss the lofty principles of each amongst themselves.

Gandhi grew to believe that just as one should love all people and all beings, one should love all faiths. Accordingly, he held the same reverence for the faiths of others as he held for his own.[49]

> *Looking at all religions with an equal eye, we would not only not hesitate but would think it our duty to blend into our faith every acceptable feature of other faiths.*
>
> Gandhi, *Yeravda Mandir* [50]

Gandhi believed that religion was a sign of humankind's humble search for meaning, and that each faith was appropriate for its own specific culture.

To Gandhi, God had been given a thousand names. Because God's qualities were infinite, God could be called by any name. God went beyond nomenclature.[51]

> *The soul of religions is one, but it is encased in a*
> *multitude of forms. Wise men will ignore the out-*
> *ward crust and see the same soul living under a*
> *variety of crusts.*
>> Gandhi, *Young India*, 25 September 1925 [52]

Gandhi felt great respect for the religious beliefs of others and believed that variations in religious perspectives were more manifestations of one's varying nation of origin, than of fundamental differences in philosophy.

> *I do not foresee a time when there would be only*
> *one religion on earth in practice. In theory, since*
> *there is only one God, there can be only one re-*
> *ligion. But in practice, no two persons I have*
> *known have had the same identical conception*
> *of God. Therefore, there will, perhaps, always be*
> *different religions answering to different temper-*
> *aments and climatic conditions.*
>> Gandhi "Some Questions Answered"
>> *Harijan*, 2 February 1934 [53]

> *God comes to us in the form in which*
> *we long to see Him.*
>> Gandhi, Letter to Raojibhai Patel,
>> 7 March 1914 [54]

THE JAIN FAITH

In describing his youth in the State of Gujarat, Gandhi states that his family, the Gandhis, was of the *Vaishnava* Hindu faith. Although they were Hindus, many of their beliefs were similar to those of Jains. Followers of the *Vaishnava* Hindu faith were usually vegetarian.

The Jain faith was strong in Gujarat. Gandhi remarked that he felt its influence everywhere and at all times. He believed that the opposition to and repulsion against eating meat was stronger in Gujarat than in any other region inside or outside of India.

This was due to the combined values of both Jain and *Vaishnava* Hindu faiths. People of both faiths believed strongly in the sanctity of all life. [55]

Those of Jain faith value the life of each and every created being. In addition to respecting the lives of humans and other large mammals, they go even one step further and respect the lives of small animals, birds, fish, tiny microbes and even sub-microscopic organisms. Jains often avoid sweet and fermented foods, and also some plants with seeds, because these may contain minute life forms, termed nigodas, that are not visible to the human eye.

With such strong principles concerning not killing, Jains object to the consumption of animal flesh, as this is integrally related to the taking of an animal's life.[56]

The first vow of Mahavira, the last great spiritual leader of the Jains, was to renounce all killing of living beings, whether human or non-human, whether large or small, whether moving or still. He vowed not to kill, not cause others to kill, and not consent to others killing any living being.[57]

Jains recognize that every creature and every being suffers pain. They believe that by inflicting harm upon any being, one has committed a sin.[58]

The Jain philosophy of nonviolence manifests its full expression during India's four-month monsoon season. During monsoon season, plant and insect life flourishes. To avoid walking on and injuring these life forms, Jains are extremely cautious and remain indoors. When they must venture outdoors, they gently brush the ground ahead of them. This concern for all beings epitomizes the essence of Jain philosophy.[59]

Gandhi did not view the Jain faith as fully distinct from Hinduism, but rather as an attempted reform of its weaker aspects.[60] He believed that his reading of the Jain scriptures had helped him tremendously along his spiritual path, because of its

> *Scrupulous regard for all things that live.*
> Gandhi, Hinduism, *The Star,* 10 March 1905 [61]

THE BUDDHIST FAITH

Gautama Siddhartha, the Buddha, was born the son of a Hindu chieftain of a hill tribe in the Shakyas, in present-day southern Nepal. During most of his life, Buddha lived and taught along the banks of the Ganges River in India. He taught that each individual must forge his or her own personal path to attain inner peace. He believed that only one who lives a life of nonviolence can attain such peace, and only when all people seek lives of nonviolence will humankind be able to secure world peace. Buddha taught people to live without inflicting harm or death upon any human or nonhuman being,[62] and to have pity on all living creatures.[63]

Ancient Buddhist scriptures tell of Buddha's desire to extend goodwill and peace to all beings, whether great or small, strong or weak, and seen or unseen.[64] The scriptures advise one not to take the life of any being, at any time, in any place, for any reason.[65]

The first vow that a Buddhist monk must make is that of vegetarianism. In many Buddhist communities, this means a total commitment to vegetarianism. In others, it means a monk may eat animal flesh, but only if the animal had not been killed specifically for that individual.[66]

Buddhist monks are advised to use a cloth to strain drinking water in order to avoid taking the life of any unseen life forms that may possibly be living within the water.[67]

Gandhi viewed Buddha as a man who was born a Hindu, was raised a Hindu, and who followed Hindu teachings. He sought to reform Hinduism, not replace it. Gandhi found the foundational principles of Buddhism and Hinduism to be identical.

Gandhi wrote that Buddha sought to teach people that one's sins could not be washed away through the blood of innocent animals sacrificed in the hope of appeasing God. Gandhi held great respect for the compassion and non-violence of Buddha, saying

> *Look at Gautama's compassion! It was not confined to mankind, it was extended to all living beings. Does not your heart overflow with love to think of the lamb being joyously perched on his shoulders?*
>
> Gandhi, *Autobiography* [68]

Buddha taught the world to treat even the lowest creatures as equal to oneself, and to hold the life of even the crawling things of the earth as precious as one's own life. He did not believe that human beings were lords and masters of the lower forms of creation, but rather, they were trustees, or protectors, of the lower animal kingdom.[69]

> *He regarded the lowest animal life as dear to his own world.*
>
> Gandhi, Speech at Public Meeting, Badulla,
> 19 November 1927 [70]

THE CHRISTIAN FAITH

Gandhi held great reverence for the teachings of Jesus and felt that Jesus' underlying message was one of non-violence towards all people and all beings. He also felt that Jesus sought to share unconditional love amongst all humanity and the entirety of creation.

The personality of Jesus held a fascination for Gandhi all his life.[71] Jesus' teachings contributed to Gandhi's faith in non-violence. He believed that millions of Christians worldwide believed likewise.

He believed that Jesus lived following the principle of *ahimsa* and possessed the faith to accept the loss of his own life unarmed and unafraid. Gandhi felt that all true followers of Jesus will not only refrain from hatred, but will also overcome evil and hate, with love and goodwill.[72]

Gandhi held the words of Jesus and of the *Bible* in great esteem, stating,

> *I have endeavored to study the Bible with the eyes of a devout Christian and I have not hesitated to assimilate whatever I have found to be good in these scriptures.*
>
> Gandhi, Speech at Public Meeting,
> Kottayam, *Harijan*, 30 January 1937 [73]

Gandhi stated that the *Bible* had been as much a book of religion to him as was the *Bhagavad Gita*.[74] He was particularly drawn to the teachings of non-violence and love in Jesus' *Sermon on the Mount*:

> *Blessed are the Merciful, for they shall obtain mercy.*
> *Blessed are the pure in heart, for they shall see God.*
> *Blessed are the peacemakers, for they shall be called sons of God.*
> *Blessed are those who are persecuted for righteousness sake, for theirs is the kingdom of heaven.*
>
> Gospel of Matthew, 5:7-10 [75]

Gandhi felt that Jesus wanted others to live, as he had, with their hearts filled with love and non-violence toward all. Gandhi believed that Jesus did not merely want others to believe in him, but to follow his ways.

> *Jesus lived and died in vain if he did not teach us to regulate the whole of life by the eternal law of love.*
>
> Gandhi, Is Non-violence Effective?
> *Harijan*, 7 January 1939 [76]

PART TWO

THE CULTIVATION

OF VALUES

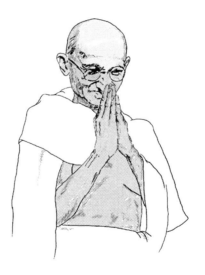

My personal faith is absolutely clear. I cannot intentionally hurt anything that lives.

*Gandhi, Letter to the Viceroy,
Lord Irwin, 2 March 1930* [1]

PART TWO

THE CULTIVATION OF VALUES

CHAPTER 4:
GANDHI'S BELIEF THAT GOD EXISTS IN ALL BEINGS

Gandhi believed it was because of his Hindu faith that he was able to perceive the breath of God pervading every fiber of every being.

> *God is neither in heaven, nor down below, but in every one.*
> Gandhi, *My God* [2]

Gandhi saw God in all that was seen and all that was unseen, and in all that was known and all that was unknown.

> *Hinduism believes in the oneness not merely of all human life but in the oneness of all that lives.*
> Gandhi, Why I am a Hindu, *Young India,*
> 20 October 1927 [3]

Based upon this, he developed his personal beliefs concerning the equality of all beings, and the right of all to live.

> *In the presence of God, the Ruler of the Universe, who pervades everything—even those whom we have called the lowest of the low—all are equal.*
> Gandhi, Speech at Aranmula,
> 20 January 1937 [4]

Gandhi could not bear to harm any living being. As a true devotee of God, he could not hate or bear ill will toward any living creature.

> *To see the universal and all-pervading spirit of Truth face to face, one must be able to love the meanest of creatures as oneself.*
>
> Gandhi, *Autobiography* [5]

To Gandhi, a true devotee of God is one who looks on all people and all beings with love and compassion, who is free from the delusion of 'I' and 'mine,' and who reduces oneself to zero. Such an individual will never harm his fellow creatures.[6]

> *The sum total of all that lives is God. We may not be God but we are of God—even as a little drop of water is of the ocean. Imagine it torn from the ocean and flung millions of miles away. It becomes helpless torn from its surroundings, and cannot feel the might and majesty of the ocean. But if some one could point out to it that it is of the ocean, its faith could revive.*
>
> Gandhi, *Harijan*, 6 March 1939 [7]

Gandhi felt an intense kinship with all beings, and believed that as humans were made in the image of God, and God protects humankind, that humankind has the responsibility to protect all other beings.

> *My ethics do not permit me to claim but require me to own kinship with not merely the ape, but the horse and the sheep, the lion and the leopard, the snake and the scorpion.*
>
> Gandhi, More Animal than Human,
> *Young India*, 8 July 1926 [8]

Gandhi felt that before human beings think they have the right to kill any being they consider venomous, they must first rid themselves of all venomous thoughts. To judge the value of a life by its outer appearance is certainly not as wise as judging it by its inner essence.

> *I do not want to live at the cost of the life, even of a snake. I should let him bite me to death rather than kill him. I believe that snakes, tigers, etc. are God's answers to the poisonous, wicked, evil thoughts we harbor. I believe all life is one. Thoughts take definite forms. Tigers and snakes have kinship with us. They are warning us to avoid harboring evil, wicked, lustful thoughts. If I want to rid myself of venomous beasts and reptiles, I must rid myself of venomous thoughts.*
>
> Gandhi, Faith vs. Reason, *Young India*,
> 14 January 1927 [9]

Universal compassion became part of Gandhi's creed. As a Hindu, he envisioned God in all beings.

> *God is omnipresent. Hence it is that He speaks to*
> *us through stones, trees, insects, birds, beasts.*
> Gandhi, *A Thought for a Day* [10]

Gandhi also envisioned God's soul flowing and integrating everything that exists in infinite space and time.

> *God is not some person outside ourselves or away*
> *from the universe. He pervades everything, and is*
> *omniscient as well as omnipotent.*
> Gandhi, *Ashram Observances in Action* [11]

To Gandhi, God's presence in all creation conferred worth upon all. Accordingly, he believed all God's creatures have as much right to live as do humans.

CHAPTER 5:
GANDHI'S PHILOSOPHY OF NON-VIOLENCE

Gandhi believed that humankind must embark upon a path of non-violence towards all people and all beings, as this is the only way that life on this planet can sustain itself.

> *I do feel that spiritual progress does demand at some stage—an inexorable demand—that we should cease to kill our fellow creatures for satisfaction of our bodily wants.*
>
> Gandhi, Speech at Meeting in Lausanne,
> 8 December 1931 [12]

To Gandhi, non-violence worked more effectively than did violence. An armed individual will naturally rely on his arms. An individual who is intentionally unarmed will rely upon an unseen Higher Power, a God, or a force of Truth.[13]

The terms Gandhi used in referring to violence and non-violence are *himsa* and *ahimsa*.

Himsa
Any act of violence in thought, word, and deed.

Ahimsa
Total nonviolence in thought, word and deed.

Gandhi understood that, "The world is bound in a chain of destruction. In other words himsa is an inherent necessity for life in the body." [14] Nevertheless, he believed one must refrain from committing any acts of *himsa* beyond that which is necessary to sustain one's existence.

To Gandhi, non-violence must not remain merely a principle to be used on a particular occasion or towards a particular group of people. It must become part of one's being.[15]

> *If we turn our eyes to the time at which history has any record down to our own time, we shall find that man has been steadily progressing towards Ahimsa. Our remote ancestors were cannibals. There came a time when they were fed up with cannibalism and they began to live on chase. Next came the time when man was ashamed of leading the life of a wandering hunter. He therefore took to agriculture and depended on mother earth for his food. Thus from being a nomad he settled down to a civilized stable life. All these are signs of progressive Ahimsa and diminished Himsa.*
>
> Gandhi, *Sevagram*, 5 August 1940 [16]

Gandhi gained much of his philosophy of non-violence from Hinduism's great literary epic, the *Bhagavad Gita*. He believed this epic embodied the essence of Hinduism and he considered it his *Bible*. [17]

Although the setting of the *Bhagavad Gita* is on a battlefield, Gandhi believed its teachings were not those of violence, but rather, the blessings of non-violence.[18] The true war being fought within the *Bhagavad Gita* is the war being fought within each individual's conscience to perform one's responsibilities and fulfill one's destiny.

The *Bhagavad Gita* demonstrated the futility of violence. At the end of the great battle, even the victors shed tears of sorrow and repentance. Victory left nothing but a legacy of misery. [19]

> *To the victors, theirs was an empty glory leaving behind only seven survivors amidst a sea of countless atrocities and millions of lost lives.*
> Gandhi, God of Love, Not War, *Harijan*,
> 5 September 1936 [20]

Although Gandhi recognized that every act of living necessitated some injury to some aspect of creation, he sought to minimize this. He considered the motive behind an action the significant factor in deciding if a specific action represented necessary "*himsa*" or selfish "*himsa.*"

> *Any act of injury done from self-interest whether amounting to killing or not, is counter to ahimsa.*
> Gandhi, Y*oung India*, 4 October 1928 [21]

When addressing his fellow citizens of India, Gandhi explained his philosophy of non-violence.

> *If you have really understood the meaning of non-violence, it should be clear to you that it is not a principle or virtue to be brought into play on a particular occasion or to be practiced with reference to a particular party. It has to become part and parcel of our being.*
> Gandhi, Talk to Khudai Khidmatgars,
> *A Pilgrimage for Peace*, 23 October 1938 [22]

Gandhi believed that one of the virtues of non-violence lay in its simplicity. By merely practicing it, one attains the ability to use it. [23]

> *Non-violence is capable of being practiced by the millions, not with full knowledge of its implications, but because it is the law of our species. It distinguishes man from the brute. [Man only] has to strive to do so.*
>
> Gandhi to the Gandhi Seva Sangh,
> *Harijan,* 4 November 1939 [24]

To Gandhi, however, a prerequisite for one to fully embody non-violence is faith in God. One must possess the strength to submit to God.

> *For me the only certain means of knowing God is non-violence-ahimsa-love.*
>
> Gandhi, *Young India*, 3 April 1924 [25]

An additional prerequisite is Truth. One who is not truthful in thought, word, and deed cannot succeed in maintaining a life of non-violence. Gandhi considered untruth, itself, a manifestation of violence.[26] One who follows a path of truth will see God within all beings.

> *To see the universal and all-pervading spirit of Truth face to face one must be able to love the meanest of creatures as oneself.*
>
> Gandhi, *Autobiography*[27]

Gandhi did not believe in using animals for humankind's selfish purposes. Hinduism taught him to value the soul in all beings equally.

> *Complete non-violence is complete absence of ill will against all that lives. It therefore embraces even subhuman life not excluding noxious insects or beasts. They have not been created to feed our destructive propensities. If we only knew the Creator, we should find their proper place in His creation.*
>
> Gandhi, *Young India*, 3 September 1922 [28]

Initially, Gandhi's non-violence had been a personal creed of ethics that included love, truth, service, considerate means, kind deeds, sincere words, tender tolerance for differences, and moderation in the pursuit of one's personal goals. Over time, it became a spiritual philosophy on a higher level.

> *The question of killing and non-killing, of man's relation to his fellow creatures, belongs to the spiritual realm. Both my intellect and heart refuse to believe that other forms of life have been created for destruction by man. God is good and wise. A good and wise God cannot be so bad and so unwise as to create to no purpose.*
>
> Gandhi, Right to Live, *Harijan*,
> 9 January 1937 [29]

To Gandhi, non-violence was the greatest force at the disposal of humankind. It was greater than the mightiest weapon of destruction designed by humankind. For one to fully embody non-violence in one's heart, however, one must first develop a foundation of religious or spiritual inner peace.

> *I believe myself to be saturated with ahimsa—*
> *non-violence. Ahimsa and truth are my two lungs.*
> *I cannot live without them. But I see every mo-*
> *ment with more and more clearness, the immense*
> *power of ahimsa and the littleness of man.*
> Gandhi, *Young India*, 21 October 1926 [30]

Gandhi believed strongly in India's practice of cow protection. He viewed the cow as a symbol of all weaker beings over which humankind possessed power. He considered it the duty of a Hindu not only to protect cows, but to protect the entire animal kingdom as well.

> *Cow protection is the dearest possession of the*
> *Hindu heart. No one who does not believe in cow*
> *protection can possibly be a Hindu. It is a noble*
> *belief. Cow worship to me means worship of in-*
> *nocence. For me, the cow is the personification of*
> *innocence. Cow protection means the protection*
> *of the weak and the helpless.*
> Gandhi, *Young India,* 8 June 1921 [31]

To Gandhi, cow protection represented protection of the entire sub-human world. He believed the cow was selected for such an honor because while she was the giver of plenty, giving milk and making agriculture possible, she harmed no one.

> *The cow is the purest form of sub-human life. She pleads for us on behalf of the whole of the sub-human species for justice to it at the hands of man, the first among all that lives. She seems to speak to us through her eye: 'You are not appointed over us to kill us and eat our flesh or otherwise ill-treat us, but to be our friend and guardian.'*
>
> Gandhi, *Young India,* 26 June 1924 [32]

Gandhi viewed Hinduism's worship of the cow as a unique contribution to the evolution of humanitarian values and toward the recognition of the sacredness of all life.[33]

> *Cow protection means the protection of the weak and the helpless. Cow protection means brotherhood between man and beast.*
>
> Gandhi, Save the Cow, *Young India,* 8 June 1921 [34]

To Gandhi, through such compassionate concern, humankind became the servant of all creation, rather than lord and master over it.

> *The cow is a poem of pity. One reads pity in the gentle animal. She is the mother to millions of Indian mankind. . . . Hinduism will continue to live so long as there are Hindus to protect the cow.*
>
> Gandhi, *Young India,* 6 October 1921 [35]

The following summarizes and explains:

Gandhi's Philosophy of Non-Violence

Non-violence is the law of the human race.

Non-violence is infinitely greater and superior to brute force.

Non-violence does not avail those who do not possess faith in a God of love.

Non-violence does not avail those who do not possess equal love for all mankind.

Non-violence affords full protection of one's self-respect and honor, but not always of one's possessions.

Non-violence is of no assistance in defense of ill-gotten gains and immoral acts.

Those seeking to practice non-violence must be prepared to sacrifice their all—except their honor.

Non-violence is a power which can be equally attainable by all.

When seeking non-violence as one's law in life, it must pervade all one's being and not be used solely for isolated acts.

Non-violence is attainable for the entirety of humankind.

Gandhi, God of Love, Not War,
Harijan, 5 September 1936 [36]

CHAPTER 6:
GANDHI'S PHILOSOPHY OF NON-ABUNDANCE

Gandhi believed that any time one takes more from the world than one needs, or unnecessarily takes the breath of life from any being, one is committing violence.

> *Not to hurt any living thing is no doubt a part of ahimsa. But it is its least expressive. The principle of ahimsa is hurt by every evil thought, by undue haste, by lying, by hatred, by wishing ill to anybody. It is also hurt by our holding on to what the world needs.*
>
> Gandhi, Ashram Vows 1930,
> From weekly discourses at Yeravda Jail [37]

Gandhi viewed true love of God as true compassion for all human and non-human beings. One with true love of God will not destroy any form of life or creation that need not be destroyed to sustain one's own existence. Gandhi did not believe one should eat a meal for simple pleasure, if by doing this, one causes the annihilation of another being.

> *Our ignorance or negligence of the Divine Law, which gives man from day to day his daily bread and no more, has given rise to inequalities with all the miseries attendant upon them.*
>
> Gandhi, Ashram Vows 1930,
> From weekly discourses at Yeravda Jail [38]

To Gandhi, any form of abundance, somehow, down a cascading chain of events, would invariably lead to the suffering of another human or non-human being.

Gandhi believed one of the main message of the *Bhagavad Gita* was renunciation. It guided people away from worldly pursuits, and taught them that one must fulfill one's allotted responsibilities, yet renounce the fruits of one's actions. When one renounces such fruits, life becomes simple. From such simplicity springs peace.[39]

> *The rich have a superfluous store of things which they do not need, and which are therefore neglected and wasted; while millions are starved to death for want of sustenance. If each retained possession only of what one needed, no one would be in want, and all would live in contentment. As it is, the rich are discontented no less that the poor.*
> Gandhi, Ashram Vows 1930,
> From weekly discourses at Yeravda Jail [40]

Gandhi believed that as civilization evolves, humankind will attain the wisdom to understand that fulfillment is attained not through material gains, but rather through spiritual ones.

> *Civilization, in the real sense of the term, consists not in the multiplication, but in the deliberate and voluntary reduction of wants. This alone promotes real happiness and contentment, and increases the capacity for service.*
> Gandhi, Ashram Vows 1930,
> From weekly discourses at Yeravda Jail [41]

To Gandhi, the solution was quite simple.

The Golden Rule is resolutely to refuse to have what millions cannot.

Gandhi, *My God* [42]

Gandhi recognized that for human civilization to sustain itself, it must depart from a path of greed and abundance. Abundance in the hands of some, invariably leads to the suffering of others—other people, other beings, and other aspects of creation.

Our civilization, our culture, our Swaraj [freedom] depends not upon multiplying our wants—self-indulgence, but upon restricting our wants—self-denial.

Gandhi, *Young India*, 6 October 1921 [43]

Gandhi believed it to be an unnecessary act of greed and abundance for humankind to rob lower animals of their lives, just to obtain a few fleeting moments of satisfaction of their palates.

As the ideals of sacrifice and simplicity were becoming more and more realized, and the religious consciousness was becoming more and more quickened in my daily life, the passion for vegetarianism as a mission went on increasing.

Gandhi, *Autobiography* [44]

Gandhi believed that when others are starving, it is a crime for one to partake of any more food than one needs.

> *It may be said without any fear of exaggeration that to partake of sweetmeats and other delicacies, in a country where the millions do not even get an ordinary full meal, is equivalent to robbery.*
>
> Gandhi, *Key to Health* [45]

Therefore, so as to prevent inflicting harm upon other people or other beings, Gandhi sought to live without excesses of any kind.

> *Unnecessary consumption is also a violation of the vow of non-violence. If, with the ideal of non-stealing in view, we reduce our consumption of things, we would grow more generous. If we do so with the ideal of non-violence, we would grow more compassionate.*
>
> Gandhi, Letter to Maganlal Gandhi,
> After 14 March 1915 [46]

Gandhi's life was his message—a message of non-violence, non-abundance, and merciful living.

When Gandhi died, his sole possessions were two pair of sandals, eating utensils, a watch given him as a gift, his eyeglasses, three holy books (the *Bhagavad Gita*, the *Bible*, and the *Koran*), and a small statue of three monkeys symbolizing, "See no evil, hear no evil, speak no evil." [47]

PART THREE

THE SPROUTING
OF BELIEFS

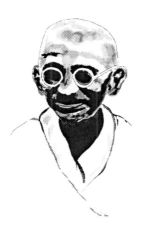

*If the body is the temple of the Holy, it re-
quires the utmost care—certainly not pam-
pering but equally certainly not disregard
or even indifference.*

Gandhi, *My Dear Child* [1]

PART THREE

THE SPROUTING OF BELIEFS

CHAPTER 7:
GANDHI'S PHILOSOPHY OF A HEALTHY LIFESTYLE

*None of us can overcome the desire to live. There
is neither sin nor shame in this desire.*
Gandhi, Letter to Ramdas Gandhi,
19 October 1934 [2]

Gandhi sought to live simply, naturally and humbly. He believed that if humankind would just live without greed and
abundance, all humanity would have the chance to live the
lifespan its Maker intended.

When reading Gandhi's views on health and nutrition, it is
important to remember that he was neither a physician nor a
dietician. Rather, he was a wise, dedicated and sincere individual, who was concerned about the welfare of his people
and who strived to live in search of truth.

His beliefs were based upon his pensive, careful observa-
tions of the lifestyles people followed, and the effects these
had on their health.

Gandhi lived at a time when little was known about health,
and even less about disease. Nevertheless, most of the
medical diagnoses he arrived at remain remarkably accu-
rate even today.

In my search after truth, I have discarded many ideas and learnt many new things. Old as I am in age, I have no feeling that I have ceased to grow inwardly or that my growth will stop at the dissolution of the flesh.

Gandhi, *Harijan*, 29 April 1933 [3]

Gandhi was a strong proponent of the philosophy that one's lifestyle had at least some effect upon one's health, and that one should consider every illness a breach of some unknown law of nature. One should strive to know the laws and pray for the ability to change and obey. One must also recognize that illness is the result not only of our actions, but also of our thoughts.[4]

Gandhi felt that a sick individual should analyze himself and try to understand the underlying causes of his illness.

[People should] *acquire a workable knowledge of the body which plays such an important part in the evolution of the soul within.*

Gandhi, *Young India*, 8 August 1929 [5]

He believed that if people humbled themselves, accepted responsibility for their own health, and sought to live simple, non-abundant, natural, and peaceful lives, they would be able to live the healthiest lives possible.

The body does not belong to us. While it lasts, we must use it as a trust handed over to our charge.

Gandhi, Ashram Vows 1930.
From weekly discourses at *Yeravda Jail* [6]

Gandhi was disillusioned by Western medicine. He felt its goal was to treat disease, not to establish health. He considered a real healer one who sought to cure people naturally, and who held a greater desired to help people maintain their health, than to treat those diseases that could have been prevented.

Gandhi did not claim that such education would confer perfect health or immortality upon any individual, but just that it would certainly help people prevent those illnesses it was in their power to prevent.

> *It is not claimed that Nature Cure can cure all disease. No system of medicine can do that or else we should all be immortals.*
> Gandhi, *Harijan*, 7 April 1946 [7]

Gandhi felt that one who seeks to understand the lifestyle that is naturally healthiest for one's body, will have a better chance of maintaining health than one who merely searches for treatments for one's ailment.

He believed in the science of natural therapy for the treatment of disease, based on the use of those natural elements which constitute the human body.[8]

> *I plea for the sake of this ancient science for a spirit of genuine search amongst Ayurvedic physicians. I am as anxious as the tallest among them can be to free ourselves from the tyranny of Western medicines which are ruinously expensive and the preparation of which takes no account of the higher humanities.*
> Gandhi, *Young India*, 8 August 1929 [9]

Gandhi considered it the duty of every individual to learn the fundamental facts concerning one's body and one's health. He considered ignorance one of the root causes of disease. To Gandhi, it was a tragedy that people did not care for their own health, and then believed that medicines could cure them.

Gandhi considered illness or disease a sign of filth that had accumulated in some portion of the mind or body. One with wisdom would clean this rather than cover it up with medicines.[10]

Although physicians treat diseases, Gandhi considered it more important that people learn how to retain their health. He was disheartened that so few physicians taught this.[11]

> *In trying to cure one old disease, we give rise to a hundred new ones.*
>
> Gandhi, *Autobiography* [12]

Gandhi felt that each individual must accept that, at least in part, their illnesses are the result of their own wrong doings. He did not teach that ailments were the karmic result of misdeeds in prior lives, but rather, that they were result of actions in one's present life.[13]

> *It is for our good to accept that our illnesses are the result of our negative thoughts and our misdeeds, and these will manifest not in a future life, but in the present one.*
>
> Gandhi, *The Bhagavad Gita* [14]

Gandhi believed that the First Law of Humanity should be, 'A healthy mind in a healthy body.' He recognized an integral relationship between mind and body, and believed that if one is healthy in one's mind, one will be able to live without violence, naturally obey the laws of nature, and naturally maintain a healthy body. He established six fundamental laws of health and hygiene:

Fundamental Laws of Hygiene and Health

1. Think the purest thoughts, and banish all idle and impure thoughts.

2. Breathe the fresh air day and night.

3. Establish a balance between bodily and mental work.

4. Stand erect, sit erect, and be neat and clean in every one of your acts, and let these be an expression of your inner condition.

5. Eat to live for service of fellow-men. Do not live for indulging yourselves. Hence, your food must be just enough to keep your mind and body in good order. Man becomes what he eats.

6. Your water, food and air must be clean, and you will not be satisfied with mere cleanliness, but you will infect your surroundings with the same three-fold cleanliness that you will desire yourselves.

Gandhi, *Gandhi's Health Guide* [15]

CHAPTER 8:
GANDHI'S PHILOSOPHY OF A HEALTHY DIET

In seeking to understand Gandhi's beliefs concerning foods, it is important to recognize that he valued the principles of non-violence, non-abundance, and merciful living, as essential to one's choice of diet. Gandhi's interests concerning diet were not predominantly issues of health, but rather issues of ethics concerning the means by which one chooses to sustain one's existence.

> *Then vegetarians* [during student days in London] *had a habit of talking of nothing but food and nothing but disease. I feel that is the worst way of going about the business.*
>
> Gandhi, *Harijan,* 20 February 1919 [16]

Initially, Gandhi was unsure if his vegetarian values were solely the result of the Hindu values he learned as a child, or values he consciously decided upon later. It was not until he was in London and read Mr. Salt's book on ethical vegetarianism that he felt his choice to live as a vegetarian was of his own free will.

> *It was Mr. Salt's book, A Plea for Vegetarianism, which showed me why, apart from hereditary habit, and apart from my adherence to a vow administered to me by my mother, it was right to be vegetarian. He showed me why it was a moral duty incumbent on vegetarians not to live upon fellow-animals.*
>
> Gandhi, *Harijan,* 20 February 1919 [17]

Gandhi considered one's choice concerning diet a moral responsibility. In the Ashrams he founded, control of one's sustenance was one of eleven vows one must swear to when becoming a member. These eleven vows were to be observed in the spirit of humility. Gandhi believed that humility was the key to peace and real joy.[18] The vows are as follows:

Eleven Vows of an Ashram Member

Non-violence
Truth
Non-stealing
Brahmacharya [Control of sexual activities]
Non-possession
Body Labor
Control of the Palate
Fearlessness on All Occasions
Equal respect for All Religions
Swadeshi [Being helpful to one's neighbor]
Sparshabhavana [Refusal to treat anyone
as an untouchable]

Gandhi, Letter to S. Ambujammal,
5 May 1935 [19]

Eating is necessary only for sustaining the body and keeping it a fit instrument for service. It must not be practiced for self-indulgence. Food must therefore be taken like medicine with self-restraint.

Gandhi, Ashram Observances,
Character and Nation Building [20]

Gandhi wrote a treatises on health and diet entitled *Key to Health*, between August 27, 1942 and December 18, 1942, when confined to the Aga Khan Palace in Poona, India. In that treatise, he described the aspects of diet he considered fundamental to one's physical, moral and spiritual health.

It is necessary to understand the meaning of the word health, before entering upon a description of the human body. In health, means body ease. He is a healthy man whose body is free from all disease; he carries on his normal activities without fatigue. Such a man should be able with ease to walk ten to twelve miles a day, and perform ordinary physical labor without getting tired. He can digest ordinary simple food. His mind and his senses are in a state of harmony and poise.

Gandhi, *Key to Health* [21]

A man with extraordinary physical strength is not necessarily healthy. He has merely developed his musculature, possibly at the expense of something else.

Gandhi, *Key to Health* [22]

Gandhi learned about diet and nutrition through both discussions with others and through his own systematic experiments on himself.

Underlying all of Gandhi's studies of nutrition, however, lay his fundamental philosophy that God is present in all beings, and that non-violence and non-abundance must be practiced within every aspect of one's life for one to maintain physical, mental, and spiritual health.

Gandhi believed it was each individual's moral responsibility to attain, and then maintain, the best state of health possible. It is one's responsibility to be of service to one's self, one's family, and one's community.

> *What is the use of the human body? Everything in the world can be used and abused. This applies to the body also. We abuse it when we use it for selfish purposes, for self-indulgence or in order to harm another.*
>
> Gandhi, *Key to Health* [23]

Gandhi's Hindu faith and its *Laws of Karma* and *Rebirth* influenced his views concerning the responsibility of each individual concerning his or her own health.

> *Man came into the world in order to pay off the [karmic] debt owed by him to it, that is to say, in order to serve God and His creation. Keeping this point of view in front of him, man acts as a guardian of his body. It becomes his duty to take such care of his body as to enable it to practice.*
>
> Gandhi, *Key to Health* [24]

CATEGORIES OF DIETS

Gandhi did not describe foods according to whether or not they were North or South Indian, Hindu or Islamic, or spicy or bland. He described them as to whether or not they were vegetarian or non-vegetarian.

> *Food can be divided into three categories: vegetarian, flesh and mixed. Flesh foods include fowl and fish. Milk is an animal product and cannot by any means be included in a strictly vegetarian diet. It serves the purpose of meat to a very large extent. In medical language it is classified as an animal food.*
>
> *Medical opinion is mostly in favor of a mixed diet, although there is a growing school, which is strongly of the opinion that anatomical and physiological evidence is in favor of man being a vegetarian. His teeth, his stomach, intestines, etc., seem to prove that nature has meant man to be vegetarian.*
>
> Gandhi, *Key to Health* [25]

To Gandhi, a purely vegetarian diet did not include milk.

> *Vegetarian diet, besides grains, pulses, edible roots, tubers and leaves, includes fruits, both fresh and dry. Dry fruit includes nuts like almonds, pistachio, walnut, etc.*
>
> Gandhi, *Key to Health* [26]

GRAINS

Gandhi sought to teach people that the most nutritious part of their grains, and all the foods derived from grains, was the husk. When the husk was removed, the individuals depending upon grains to help them maintain their health would suffer.

> *The richest part of wheat is contained in its bran. There is a terrible loss of nutrition when the bran wheat is removed. The villagers and others who eat whole-wheat flour ground in their own chakkis* [grinders] *save their money and, what is most important, their health.*
> Gandhi, *Harijan*, 1 February 1935 [27]

Gandhi also believed that people should eat only one grain at a time, and not mix grains. He taught that a meal consisting only of grains was not totally healthy, and should be combined with vegetables, such as onion, carrots, radish, salad leaves or tomatoes.[28]

CEREALS

Gandhi begins his *Key to Health* by discussing cereals. In Western culture, these are rarely discussed. Cereals include dishes made from wheat, rice, and other grains. They supply carbohydrates and vitamins that have sustained humanity for centuries. Gandhi did not believe in mixing cereals, or any foods for that matter. He believed it was better for one's health and discipline not to ingest more than three tastes during the same meal.

> *Different cereals are used in different provinces of India. In many places, more than one kind of cereal are eaten at the same time, for instance, small quantities of wheat, bajri and rice are served together. This mixture is not necessary for the nourishment of the body. It makes it difficult to regulate the quantity of food intake, and puts an extra strain upon digestion. As all these varieties supply starch mainly, it is better to take one only, at a time. Wheat may well be described as the king among the cereals.*
>
> Gandhi, *Key to Health* [29]

> *The cereals should be properly cleansed, ground on a grinding stone, and the resulting flour served as it is. Sieving of the rice should be avoided. It is likely to remove the bhusi, or the pericarp, which is a rich source of salts and vitamins, both of which are most valuable from the point of view of nutrition. The pericarp also supplies roughage, which helps the action of the bowels.*
>
> Gandhi, *Key to Health* [30]

RICE

Rice has remained a dietary staple for the populace of India for centuries. Gandhi's concern was that the process of polishing rice, to make it white in color and softer in consistency, was robbing the rice, and therefore the people, of all of its nutrients.

Rice should not be polished at all.
> Gandhi, Letter to Ambujammal,
> 5 May 1935 [31]

Whole, unpolished rice . . . is the most nutritious and, naturally, the cheapest.
> Gandhi, *Harijan*, 25 January 1935 [32]

Rice grain, being very delicate, has been provided by nature with an outer covering or epicarp. This is not edible. In order to remove this inedible portion, rice has to be pounded. Pounding should be just sufficient to remove the epicarp or the outer skin of the rice grain. But machine pounding not only removes the outer skin, but also polishes the rice by removing its pericarp. The explanation of the popularity of polished rice lies in the fact that polishing helps preservation. The pericarp is very sweet and unless it is removed, rice is easily attacked by certain organisms. Polished rice and wheat without its pericarp, supply us with almost pure starch. Important constituents of the cereals are lost with the removal of the pericarp.
> Gandhi, *Key to Health* [33]

PULSES
PEAS AND BEANS

The term "pulses' refers to the edible seed of many plants, or what is known in the West as peas and beans. Gandhi recognized that many people found these difficult to digest. Hence, he did not necessarily advise these for people who lived sedentary lives or who obtained protein from other sources, such as dairy.

> *Almost everybody thinks that pulses are an essential constituent of the diet. Even meat eaters must have pulses. It is easy to understand that those who have to do hard manual work and who cannot afford to drink milk, cannot do without pulses. But I can say without any hesitation whatsoever that those who follow sedentary occupations as for instance, clerks, businessmen, lawyers, doctors, teachers, and those who are not too poor to buy milk, do not require pulses. Pulses are generally considered to be difficult to digest and are eaten in much smaller quantities than cereals. Out of the varieties of pulses, peas, gram and haricot beans are considered to be the most difficult to digest, and mung and masoor (lentils) the least difficult to digest.*
>
> Gandhi, *Key to Health* [34]

Gandhi felt that, in general, pulses should be eaten sparingly.[35] He also believed that if one is consuming milk, then it is unnecessary, and also a harmful excess, to consume pulses. He felt that one who consumes dairy gets all the protein one needs from milk, and it is not necessary to consume pulses.[36]

Although Gandhi had no objection to the ingestion of uncooked pulses, he noted that in general, pulses had a tendency to cause constipation.[37]

He observed that oftentimes, those who had recently converted to vegetarianism are advised to eat pulses, butter, cheese and milk in greater quantities than they did while eating meat. Gandhi considered this a mistake.[38]

Gandhi considered soy beans to be the most nutritious beans, stating that the soy bean stands at the top of all known articles of food because of its low percentage of carbohydrates and high percentage of salts, protein and fat.[39]

VEGETABLES

Gandhi thought highly of the capabilities of the plant world
to sustain human life and health.

> *The unlimited capacity of the plant world to sus-*
> *tain man at his highest is a region yet unexplored*
> *by modern medical science.*
>> Gandhi, *Young India*, 18 July 1929 [40]

Gandhi praised the virtues of vegetables.

> *It is necessary, therefore, to correct the error that*
> *vegetarianism has made us weak in mind or body*
> *or passive or inert in action.*
>> Gandhi, *Young India*, 7 October 1926 [41]

Nevertheless, Gandhi wished that people would consume
vegetables in their natural, raw states so as to obtain the
maximum nutritional benefit from their natural supply of
vitamins.

Gandhi noted that consumption of a small quantity of vegetables, such as cucumber, pumpkins, squash, in their uncooked state was of greater benefit than consumption of
larger quantities of the same cooked. But the digestion of
many people, due to years of eating only cooked foods, had
been so impaired, that they had difficulty tolerating raw
vegetables.

Gandhi advised people that to ingest vegetables in their raw state, they must masticate well. He noted that proper chewing of foods enables one to absorb more nutrients and to sustain one's existence even when consuming smaller quantities of food, thereby:

> *Reducing the dietetic himsa that one commits to sustain life.*
>> Gandhi, *Young India*, 15 November 1928 [42]

A diet consisting of vegetables in their raw state is beneficial because

> *The addition of green leaves to their meals will enable villagers to avoid many diseases from which they are now suffering.*
>> Gandhi, *Harijan*, 15 February 1935 [43]

He advised people to consume leafy vegetables every day, and if possible, in their raw state.

> *Among fresh vegetables, a fair amount of leafy vegetables must be taken every day. I do not include potatoes, sweet potatoes, suran, etc., which supply mainly starch, among vegetables. They should be put down in the same category as starch supplying cereals.*
>
> *A fair helping of ordinary fresh vegetables is advisable. Certain varieties such as cucumber, tomatoes, mustard greens and cress and other tender leaves need not be cooked. They should be washed properly and then eaten raw in small quantities.*
>> Gandhi, *Key to Health* [44]

Gandhi deduced that whether from the viewpoint of nutrition or of *ahimsa*, the use of uncooked vegetables in one's diet is highly beneficial, stating "The ethical value of uncooked foods is incomparable." [45]

Gandhi did not try to convert others to vegetarianism, for matters of health.

> *I am not going to tell you, as I see and wander about the world, that vegetarians, on the whole, enjoy better health than meat-eaters. . . I think that what vegetarians should do is not emphasize the physical consequences of vegetarianism, but to explore the moral consequences.*
> Gandhi, *Harijan*, 20 February 1919 [46]

He believed that if one does decide to become vegetarian, one should do so for altruistic reasons, not for one's personal gain.

> *I notice also that it is those persons who become vegetarians because they are suffering from some disease or other—that is, from purely the health point of view—it is those persons who largely fall back. I discovered that for remaining staunch to vegetarianism a man requires a moral basis.*
> Gandhi, *Harijan*, 20 February 1919 [47]

It is the spirit in man for which we are concerned. Therefore vegetarians should have a moral basis—that a man was not born a carnivorous animal, but born to live on the fruits and herbs that the earth grows. . . The basis of my vegetarianism is not physical, but moral.

Gandhi, *Harijan*, 20 February 1919 [48]

FRUIT

Gandhi was particularly fond of fruits. He actually lived on a diet consisting solely of fruit for extended periods of time. He tells of a time during which he lived exclusively on fruits for six months. He consumed neither milk nor curds [yogurt] during that time.

Although he admits that six months was not a long period of time, he still observed that he was able to maintain good health, and even resist infections when others had not. After that time period, he was not able to lift heavy loads, but he perceived his general physical and mental powers to be greater than before. He also observed that he was able to function mentally with greater persistence and concentration.[49]

> *All the literature I have read points to fruits and nuts with only a small quantity of green vegetables as a perfect food.*
> Gandhi, *Young India*, 22 August 1929 [50]

Yet over the years, Gandhi modified his beliefs concerning fruits as he recognized that only small quantities of fruit were necessary on a daily basis for one to maintain optimum health.

> *Fresh fruit is good to eat, but only a little is necessary.*
> Gandhi, *Harijan*, 25 January, 1942 [51]

Gandhi advised people to consume those fruits that grow naturally during the season in which they are being consumed. He also advised people to eat fruits endogenous to the region in which they were living.

> *As for fruits, our daily diet should include the available fruits of the season, e.g., mangos, jambu, guavas, grapes, papayas, limes—sweet or sour, oranges, moosambi, etc., should be used in their season. The best time for taking fruit is in the early morning. A breakfast of fruit and milk should give full satisfaction. Those who take an early lunch may well have a breakfast of fruit only. Banana is a good fruit. But as it is rich in starch, it takes the place of bread. Milk and banana make a perfect meal.*
>
> Gandhi, *Key to Health* [52]

In addition to the general statement that one should include fresh fruits in one's diet, Gandhi considered it advisable for one to drink water containing lime juice daily.

> *Fresh fruit according to one's taste and purse. In any case it is good to take two sour limes a day. The juice should be squeezed and taken with vegetables or in water, cold or hot.*
>
> Gandhi, *Key to Health* [53]

FATS
OIL, BUTTER, GHEE

Gandhi recognized that people require a certain amount of fat in their diet. During the initial phase of Gandhi's study of foods, however, science was unaware of the health dangers of consuming fats obtained from dairy and meat.

A certain amount of fat is necessary. This can be had in the form of ghee or oil. If ghee can be had, oil becomes unnecessary. It is difficult to digest and not as nourishing as pure ghee. An ounce and a half of ghee per day, should be considered ample to supply the needs of the body. Among oils, sweet oil, ground nut oil and cocoa-nut oil should be given preference. Oil must be fresh. If available, it is better to use hand-pressed oil.

Gandhi, *Key to Health* [54]

During Gandhi's younger years, nothing was known of cholesterol and atherosclerosis. Therefore, he considered ghee, a liquefied form of butter made from cow's milk, a totally healthy food. Eventually, however, he stated

We have tentatively dropped ghee from our menu, except for those who consider it necessary for their health. We are issuing the equivalent in weight of pure vegetable oils.

Gandhi, *Harijan*, 2 November 1935 [55]

Years later, after Gandhi progressed further along in his study of dietetics, dishonest people had begun making a counterfeit form of ghee from the leaves of flowers, fruits and vegetables. This was termed *Vanaspati Ghee*. Gandhi said that *Vanaspati* was not, and could never be considered, ghee.

> *If ever it were to become ghee, I would be first loudly to proclaim that there is no further need for real ghee. Ghee or butter is the fat content of milk drawn from an animal.*
> Gandhi, *Harijan*, 14 April 1946 [56]

Yet he was more concerned about the deceptive selling of vegetable oil in the name of ghee to the Indian people. He considered it totally dishonest. Gandhi believed that this deception had led to a lack of energy, and an increase in mortality amongst those people who could not obtain sufficient nutrition any other way. He condemned such deception being inflicted upon people concerning their foods, and as a result, their health.

MILK

Gandhi's deep rooted moral and ethical values told him that humankind's ingestion of milk after the age of infancy was not necessary.

It is my firm conviction that man need take no milk at all, beyond the mother's milk that he takes as a baby.

Gandhi, *Autobiography* [57]

In my opinion there are definite drawbacks in taking milk or meat. In order to get meat we have to kill. And we are certainly not entitled to any other milk except the mother's milk of our infancy. Over and above the moral drawbacks, there are others, purely from the point of view of health. Both milk and meat bring with them the defects of the animal from which they are derived. Domesticated cattle are hardly ever healthy. Just like man, cattle suffer from innumerable diseases. Several of these are overlooked even when cattle are subjected to periodical medical examinations.

Gandhi, *Key to Health* [58]

Gandhi relays the story of when he found himself obliged to abandon his conviction that there was no need for an adult to drink milk. He had been on campaign in Kheda. Because of what he believed to have been an error in diet, he found himself critically ill. He tried to regain his health without consuming milk by consuming mung water, almond-milk, and various oils. All attempts were in vain.

This incident occurred in 1917. It was during a time when Gandhi had succumbed to severe dysentery. He felt that his illness had been caused by his own ignorance in maintaining his health.

Gandhi had made a vow never to consume cow's or buffalo's milk. While he was critically ill, however, his friends coaxed him into drinking milk obtained from another species of mammal, a goat, stating that his vow did not relate to milk from goats.

Although Gandhi knew that the spirit of the vow meant that he would never consume milk from any species, his longing to live was so strong, that he sublimated in his mind that the vow did not refer to goat's milk. He began to drink goat's milk. His conscience, however, told him that the spirit of his vow had been destroyed.[59]

> *I was reduced to a skeleton, but I stubbornly refused to take any medicine and with equal stubbornness refused to take milk or buttermilk. I could not build up my body and pick up sufficient strength to leave the bed. I had taken a vow of not taking milk. A medical friend suggested that at the time of taking the vow, I could have had in mind only the milk of a cow or buffalo; why should that vow prevent me from taking goat's milk. Goat's milk was produced immediately and I drank it. It seemed to bring me new life. I picked up rapidly and was soon able to leave the bed.*
>
> Gandhi, *Key to Health* [60]

Gandhi had always been in favor of a purely vegetarian diet, without milk.

> *I have always been in favor of a pure vegetarian diet. But experience has taught me that in order to be perfectly fit, a vegetarian diet must include milk and milk products such as curds, butter, ghee, etc. This is a significant departure from my original idea. I excluded milk from my diet for six years. At that time, I felt none the worse for the denial.*
>
> Gandhi, *Key to Health* [61]

Because of this experience, however, Gandhi was forced to humble himself and admit, at least concerning himself, the need to add milk to a strictly vegetarian diet.

> *Though my belief in the possibility of avoiding milk and ghee without endangering health is un-shakable, I cannot claim as yet to have found a combination of vegetarian foods that will invariably produce the results claimed today for milk.*
>
> Gandhi, Y*oung India*, 18 July 1929 [62]

Nevertheless, Gandhi believed that were one to search further, one would be able to find a substitute from the vegetable kingdom for milk.

> *I am convinced that in the vast vegetable kingdom there must be some kind, which, while supplying those necessary substances which we derive from milk and meat, is free from their drawbacks, ethical and other.*
>
> Gandhi, *Key to Health* [63]

Gandhi, having humbled himself with the admonition that a purely vegetarian [a vegan] diet was not sufficient to sustain his health and that he required milk, stated:

It would appear as if man is really unable to sustain life without either meat or milk or milk products.

Gandhi, *Harijan*, 13 October, 1946 [64]

Subsequent to this, for the remainder of his life, Gandhi kept his goat with him. Hence, he was able to maintain his source of milk while ensuring that no abuse was inflicted upon the animal supplying it.

I have no choice. I can find no plant or herb which can equal milk in food value. There is certainly some truth in the belief that milk is a wholesome food even for yogis. It is the only substitute for meat. Only our vaids [Ayurvedic Physicians] could have discovered a vegetable substitute for milk, but lacking zeal for the dharma, they made no such attempt. I have failed in my search and have given up.

Gandhi, Letter to D. B. Kalelkar and
B. D. Kalelkar, 19 February 1933 [65]

Gandhi, however, remained firm in his conviction that children must be supplied with milk.

> *Children should not go without milk.*
>> Gandhi, *Nature Cure* [66]

In his search for a food or foods that could adequately supply his family and himself with the same nutrients that milk supplied, he remained unsuccessful. He asked for guidance in his search for such a food.

> *In the limitless vegetable kingdom there is an effective substitute for milk, which, every medical man admits, has its drawbacks and which is designed by nature not for man but for babies and young ones of lower animals. I should count no cost too dear for making a search which in my opinion is so necessary from more points of view than one. I therefore still seek information and guidance from kindred spirits.*
>> Gandhi, *Young India,* 22 August 1929 [67]

Gandhi would certainly be happy to know the answer to this today: Soy milk!

EGGS

Gandhi ate eggs. He recognized that to some vegetarians, consumption of eggs was not acceptable. But at the time that Gandhi lived, he had no objection to consuming them.

An innocuous egg is one from which no chick can come out. Personally, I regard such eggs as acceptable food.

Gandhi, Letter to Bal Kalelkar,
12 February 1933 [68]

To Gandhi, an 'innocuous egg' was one that although having been passed by the hen, was not the result of the hen having been mated with a rooster. Hens lay eggs on a regular basis, just as women ovulate. These eggs are similar to those microscopic unfertilized eggs that a woman passes each month during the time of ovulation. Just as a women sheds these microscopic eggs along with the blood of her menstrual period each month, the hen lays her eggs on a cyclic basis as well.

These unfertilized eggs laid by hens could never produce a chicken. The hens used for egg production are kept in different locations than the roosters, but their eggs must come out no matter what. They are only mated when breeders want to produce more hens. Although unfertilized eggs outwardly appear similar to fertilized eggs, a fertilized egg can be recognized by a red blood spot within the yolk portion of the egg.

One must remember that Gandhi lived prior to the time artificial insemination of hens, used in the breeding of future hens, had become the norm. Hence, during that era consumption of eggs did not indirectly lead to the mass scale destruction of newborn male chicks at birth. Presently, very few male newborn chicks are permitted to live. They are not needed.

That is because only a very small number of roosters are needed to artificially inseminate the breeding hens used to produce future hens. This insemination is permitted only when a breeder requires new hens because the old hens are no longer manufacturing unfertilized eggs at maximum capacity, or because they need more hens for human consumption as chicken. Hence, Gandhi's decision to consume eggs was not, at that time, as morally offensive as it might be considered today.

> *From a religious point of view, they are an unnecessary addition to the number of articles which we eat, and from the point of view of vegetarianism, they are as objectionable as milk. Probably it gives a hen greater pain to carry such eggs and be caged for their sake than it does a cow to be milked. However, such eggs are not in the same category as meat, which we regard as forbidden.*
> Gandhi, Letter to Bal Kalelkar,
> 12 February 1933 [69]

SUGAR

Gandhi was not against the consumption of sugar. He did, however, feel that the quantity of sugar many people consumed was excessive for the maintenance of optimum health.

> *A certain amount of sugar is also necessary. Although sweet fruits supply plenty of sugar, there is no harm in taking one to one and a half ounces of sugar, brown or white, each day. If one cannot obtain sweet fruits, sugar may become a necessity. But the undue prominence given to sweet things nowadays is wrong. City folk eat too much of sweet things. Milk puddings, milk sweets and sweets of other kinds are consumed in large quantities. They are all unnecessary and are harmful except when taken in very small quantities.*
>
> Gandhi, *Key to Health* [70]

Gandhi believed it is better for one to consume sugars in their natural state, within the fruit from which they naturally occur, than in their processed state.

> *Sugars are best obtained from raisins, figs or dates, all of which should be taken in moderation.*
>
> Gandhi, *Young India,* 18 July 1929 [71]

CONDIMENTS

Gandhi recognized that common salt was essential to one's health. Other than salt, however, he believed people should limit their intake of condiments so as to permit the natural taste of foods to be appreciated.

> *Common salt may be rightly counted as the king among condiments. Many people cannot eat their food without it. The body requires certain salts and common salt is one of them. It might be supplemented in small quantities.*
>
> Gandhi, *Key to Health* [72]

> *Several condiments are not required by the body as a general rule, e.g., chillies, fresh or dry, pepper, turmeric, coriander, caraway, mustard, methi, asafetida, etc. These are taken just for satisfaction of the palate. My opinion, based on my own experience over fifty years, is that not one of these is needed to keep perfectly healthy.*
>
> Gandhi, *Key to Health* [73]

Gandhi also felt that too much time was spent on the preparation of food in India, and this had negatively impacted upon the intellectual role women might otherwise have played in society. He felt that because women were required to spend so much time preparing food and grinding spices, that they were missing out on other meaningful, fulfilling professions.

TEA, COFFEE, COCOA

Gandhi firmly believed that tea, coffee, and cocoa were not required by the body. He stated that the origin of tea was not for purposes of health, but rather for purposes of sanitation.

Tea originated in China. It was first employed to help people ensure the purity of their drinking water. Boiling of water was essential to make it safe for consumption. Someone discovered a form of grass called 'tea,' which when added to water would turn a golden color as the water reached the boiling point. After this discovery, people began adding tea leaves to their water to confirm it had been adequately boiled.

Gandhi went on to say, however, that tea, as it is commonly consumed, is actually harmful.

> *The leaves contain tannin which is harmful to the body. Tannin is generally used in Tanneries to harden leather. When taken internally it produces a similar effect upon the mucous lining of the stomach and intestine. This impairs digestion and causes dyspepsia.*
> Gandhi, *Key to Health*, 18 December 1942 [74]

Gandhi notes that habitual tea drinkers begin to feel restless if they do not consume their cup at the usual time. He also states that what is said about tea applies more or less to coffee as well. Gandhi quotes a Hindustani saying about coffee:

Coffee allays cough and relieves flatulence, but it impairs physical and sexual vigor and makes the blood watery, so that there are three disadvantages against its two advantages. I do not know how far the saying is justified. I hold a similar opinion with regard to cocoa.

Gandhi, *Key to Health*, 18 December 1942 [75]

Gandhi said that he used to suffer from all sorts of ailments, one after the other when he was drinking any of these beverages (tea, coffee, cocoa). Then, when he gave them up he lost nothing, and felt he had benefited a great deal. He could get the same sense of fulfillment from clear vegetable soup that he had previously derived from tea and the other beverages. He was able to substitute these with total satisfaction and to maintain health by drinking hot water, honey, and lemon.[76]

ALCOHOL

Gandhi was totally against the use of intoxicants of any kind.

> *There is a school who favor limited and regulated consumption of alcohol and believe it to be useful. I have not found any weight in their argument.*
> Gandhi, *Key to Health*, 9 October 1942 [77]

According to Gandhi, all forms of liquor should be strictly avoided. Any advantages to be gained from ingestion of these are available through other forms of sustenance. He felt that alcohol made an individual incapable of doing anything useful.

> *Those who take to drinking ruin themselves and their people. They lose all sense of decency and propriety.*
> Gandhi, *Key to Health*, 9 October 1942 [78]

Gandhi related stories of people from a variety of cultures who fell victim to the habit of alcohol ingestion and ended their lives in pathetic conditions. He stated

> *Alcohol ruins one physically, morally, intellectually, and economically.*
> Gandhi, *Key to Health*, 9 October 1942 [79]

ANIMAL FLESH

It was Gandhi's strong personal conviction that when human beings consume the flesh of other beings:

> *We kill ourselves, our body and soul.*
> Gandhi, *Moral Basis of Vegetarianism* [80]

He had come to this realization through a combination of both his Hindu religious and cultural values, and his natural inclination toward such beliefs.

> *By instinct and upbringing I personally favor a purely vegetarian diet.*
> Gandhi, *Young India*, 15 August 1929 [81]

In discussing the philosophy of vegetarianism in India, Gandhi explained that the great majority of people in India are vegetarians, some because of religious convictions and others because they cannot afford to buy meat.

Yet even those who consider themselves meat-eaters, do not believe they need to consume meat to remain healthy or that they will die without meat.[82] Gandhi said that meat-eaters in India do not generally regard meat as a necessity, but generally take it as a side dish along with their grain dishes.[83]

Gandhi believed that examination of the structure of the human body leads one to the conclusion that humans were meant to live on vegetarian diets. He notes the close affinity between the internal organs of humans and the organs of other fruit-eating animals, such as the monkey, noting that its teeth and stomach are similar to those of humans.

He then considers the organs of carnivorous animals, such as the lion and tiger, and notes that their teeth and stomach are totally different from those of humans. Because of this, scientists have determined that humankind was not intended to sustain its existence on meat, but rather on roots and fruits.[84]

Gandhi's strongest objections to the consumption of meat were moral ones. Nevertheless, he considered health objections to be significant as well. He noted that both milk and meat carry with them the defects of the animal from which they are derived, and that domesticated animals are rarely of perfect health.[85]

To Gandhi, there was no question as to whether or not human beings required meat to maintain their strength and their health. They just did not! To Gandhi, adoption of a vegetarian diet had been a priceless gift. It helps one advance in one's spiritual progress.[86]

> *Unless the mind and the body and the soul are made to work in unison, they cannot be adequately used for the service of mankind. Physical, mental and spiritual purity is essential for their harmonious working.*
>
> Gandhi, *Bhagavad Gita* [87]

Although Gandhi was certain that ingestion of flesh was disadvantageous to one's health, he recognized that the large and powerful industries involved in the production of meat would hinder the medical profession from bringing such information to the public.

> *The tremendous vested interests that have grown around the belief in animal food prevent the medical profession from approaching the question with complete detachment. It almost seems to me that it is reserved for lay enthusiasts to cut their way through a mountain of difficulties even at the risk of their lives to find the truth.*
>
> Gandhi, *Young India*, 15 August 1929 [88]

In discussing non-vegetarian dietary practices of a large portion of humanity, Gandhi stated

> *We are not ashamed to sacrifice a multitude of other lives in decorating the perishable body and trying to prolong its existence for a few fleeting moments with the result that we kill ourselves, both body and soul.*
>
> Gandhi, *Autobiography*, [89]

Decades ago, without concrete evidence that ingestion of animal flesh was harmful to the health of human beings, Gandhi came to his unswerving convictions, that,

> *I do not regard flesh-food as necessary for us at any stage and under any climate in which it is possible for human beings ordinarily to live. I hold flesh-food to be unsuitable to our species. We err in copying the lower animal world if we are superior to it. Experience teaches that animal food is unsuitable to those who would curb their passions.*
>
> Gandhi, *Young India*, 7 October 1926 [90]

Gandhi hoped that humankind would recognize the violence involved in the act of obtaining animal flesh for consumption, and gradually orient itself towards vegetarian lifestyles.

> *He whose eyes are opened to the truth of violence in beef-eating or meat-eating, and has therefore rejected them, who loves 'both man and bird and beast' is worthy of our adoration.*
>
> Gandhi, *Young India*, 5 April 1926 [91]

Gandhi's convictions underlying his decision to live without consuming the flesh of animals is expressed in his one simple statement:

> *In order to get meat, we have to kill.*
>
> Gandhi, *Key to Health* [92]

We serve the good of the world by refraining from causing suffering to them, because we shall refrain from doing so only if we cherish the lives of other creatures as we do our own.

Gandhi, *The Bhagavad Gita* [93]

FREQUENCY OF MEALS

Gandhi believed that people should discipline themselves to eat three times a day rather than to nibble all day.

> *How often should one eat? Many people take two meals a day. The general rule is to take three meals: breakfast early in the morning and before going out to work, dinner at midday and supper in the evening or later. There is no necessity to have more than three meals. In the cities some people keep on nibbling from time to time. This habit is harmful. The digestive apparatus requires rest.*
>
> Gandhi, *Key to Health* [94]

Basically, Gandhi believed that people should not eat too often or too much. He felt they should consider consumption of food a responsibility to sustain their health, rather than a luxury to appease their palate.

> *Now let us consider how often and how much should one eat. Food should be taken as a matter of duty—even as a medicine—to sustain the body, never for the satisfaction of the palate. By acting thusly, pleasurable feeling comes from satisfaction of real hunger.*
>
> Gandhi, *Key to Health* [95]

QUANTITY OF FOOD

One of Gandhi's main beliefs concerning ingestion of food was that one must limit one's intake just to the amount needed to sustain the health of the body. One should eat to ensure that mind and body can function in health and ease, and not eat merely for enjoyment.

> *About nothing are we so woefully negligent or ignorant as in regard to our bodies. Instead of using the body as a temple of God we use it as a vehicle of indulgences.*
>
> Gandhi, *Young India*, 8 August 1929 [96]

Gandhi believed in living a life of simplicity and in eating sparingly. He believed that those who spend their days in devotion to God understand that eating a full meal every day is a hindrance to one's life of devotion.[97]

The following is a list of the types and quantities of food Gandhi considered healthy for a sedentary individual to consume daily:[97]

Cereals (wheat, rice, bajri, etc.)	6 oz.
Vegetables leafy	3 oz.
Vegetables others	5 oz.
Vegetables raw	1 oz.
Ghee	1 ½ oz.
or Butter	2 oz.
Gur or white sugar	1 ½ oz.
Cow's milk	1 to 2 quarts

Gandhi held a firm conviction that

> *For the seeker who would live in fear of God and who would see Him face to face, restraint in diet both as to quantity and quality is as essential as restraint in thought and speech.*
>
> Gandhi, *Autobiography* [99]

Gandhi observed that even though an individual might be vegetarian, that did not mean that the individual had attained the ability to control the quantity of food consumed.

> *I found also that several vegetarians found it impossible to remain vegetarians because they had made food a fetish and because they thought that by becoming vegetarians they could eat as much lentils, haricot beans, and cheese as they liked. Of course these people could not possibly keep their health.*
>
> Gandhi, *Harijan*, 20 February 1919 [100]

> *I discovered that in order to keep health, no matter what you ate, it was necessary to cut down the quantity of the food, and reduce the number of meals. Become moderate; err on the side of less, rather than on the side of more. When I invite friends to share their meals with me I never press them to take anything except only what they require. On the contrary, I tell them not to take a thing if they do not want it.*
>
> Gandhi, *Harijan*, 20 February 1919 [101]

Although Gandhi taught people to limit the quantity of foods they consumed to that amount necessary to maintain health, he did not believe one should limit one's diet to such an extent that one can no longer be of use to society. One who did that would no longer be making full use of the instrument that God had placed at one's disposal.

> *One should make do with the fewest possible articles* [of food] *and in the smallest possible quantity, no more than is absolutely necessary to pay the body its hire. It will be best to frame the rules of our diet bearing this principle in mind.*
>
> Gandhi, Letter to Jamnadas Gandhi,
> 17 March 1914 [102]

> *Mortification of the flesh is a necessity when the flesh rebels against one; it is a sin when the flesh has come under subjection and can be used as an instrument of service. In other words, there is no inherent merit in mortification of the flesh.*
>
> Gandhi, *Harijan*,
> 2 November 1935 [103]

SELF-RESTRAINT

Gandhi believed that one who exercised no restraint in one's intake of foods had become a slave to one's animal passions.

> *One who has not been able to control his palate,*
> *will never be able to control the other senses.*
> Gandhi, *Key to Health*, 13 December 1942 [104]

He believed that one should take just enough food for the essential needs of the body and no more.

> *Because of our incorrect habits and artificial*
> *way of living, very few people know what their*
> *system requires. Our parents who bring us into*
> *this world do not, as a rule, cultivate self-control.*
> *Their habits and their way of living influence*
> *children to a certain extent.*
> Gandhi, *Key to Health* [105]

The diet should be healthy and well-balanced, and, the body should not become a slave to the demands of the palate. Habits of self-restraint should be cultivated.

> *My experience teaches me that, for those whose*
> *minds are working towards self-restraint, dietetic*
> *restrictions and fasting are very helpful.*
> Gandhi, *Autobiography* [106]

*One should eat not in order to please the palate
but just to keep the body going. When each organ
of sense subserves the body and through the body
the soul . . . then alone does it begin to function in
the way nature intended it to do.*

Gandhi, *Autobiography* [107]

Gandhi noted that self-restraint, once cultivated, would become a matter of habit.

*Habits once formed are difficult to shed. There are
very few who succeed in getting rid of them. But
when the realization comes to an individual that
he is his own bodyguard, and his body has been
dedicated to service, he desires to learn laws of
keeping his body in a fit condition and tries hard
to follow them.*

Gandhi, *Key to Health* [108]

And, once self-restraint has been cultivated, it is beneficial to one's soul.

*Morally, I have no doubt that a diet of self-denial
is good for the soul. The diet of a man of self-
restraint must be different from that of a man of
pleasure, just as their ways of life must be different.*

Gandhi, *Autobiography* [109]

FASTING

Gandhi was a strong proponent of fasting. He valued it as an act of physical and spiritual sacrifice.

> *A genuine fast cleanses body, mind and soul. It crucifies the flesh and to that extent sets the soul free. A sincere prayer can work wonders. It is an intense longing of the soul for its even greater purity. Purity thus gained when it is utilized for a noble purpose becomes a prayer.*
> Gandhi, *Young India,* 24 March 1920 [110]

Gandhi believes it is necessary for one to learn control of one's senses. To enter into and maintain a fast, one must cultivate three traits: faith, control of the senses, and recognition that excesses cause harm.

> *Fasting is futile unless it is accompanied by an incessant longing for self-restraint.*
> Gandhi, *Autobiography* [111]

Gandhi observed that, in many people, the instinctive pleasure for food did not always stop when the body had enough. He advised such individuals to pray to God for assistance in restraining their diet.

> *If physical fasting is not accompanied by mental fasting, it is bound to end up in hypocrisy and disaster.*
> Gandhi, *Autobiography* [112]

He believed that when eating ceases to serve the fundamental purpose of nourishing the body, it should be limited. Just as when steam fails to make an engine run, its supply ought to be stopped, so too should food intake be halted when it is no longer needed to sustain one's body.

> *Fasting and restriction in diet now play an important part in my life. Passion in man is generally coexistent with a hankering after the pleasures of the palate. And so it was with me. If I had failed to develop restraint to the extent that I have, I should have descended lower than the beasts and met my doom long ago.*
>
> Gandhi, *Autobiography* [113]

Gandhi believed that a fast should last for ten to twenty days, or longer. He recognized that one's attainment of pleasure from food is difficult to conquer, but one should not accept defeat in one's attempts to control one's diet. If one fails, one should simply start one's fast again. Even if one fails ten or twenty times, if one perseveres, one will ultimately succeed.[114]

> *Observing, I saw that a man should eat sparingly and now and then fast. No man or woman really ate sparingly or consumed just that quantity which the body requires and no more. We easily fall prey to the temptations of the palate, and therefore when a thing tastes delicious we do not mind taking a morsel or two more. But you cannot keep health under those circumstances.*
>
> Gandhi, *Harijan*, 20 February 1919 [115]

TOLERANCE FOR NON-VEGETARIANS

Addressing his fellow vegetarians of India, predominantly of Hindu, Buddhist and Jain faiths, Gandhi beseeched them to have tolerance for those of other faiths who were not vegetarian.

The golden rule of conduct is mutual tolerance, seeing that we will never all think alike and we shall see truth in fragment and from different angles of vision.
Gandhi, *Young India*, 23 September 1926 [116]

He taught people that one cannot be too righteous concerning one's diet, or in any of one's actions, in dealing with those of other belief systems because

In life it is impossible to eschew violence completely. The question arises, where is one to draw the line? The line cannot be the same for everyone. Although the principle is essentially the same, yet everyone applies it to his or her own way. What is one man's food can be another's poison. Meat-eating is a sin for me. Yet, for another person, who has always lived on meat and never seen anything wrong with it, to give it up simply in order to copy me will be a sin.
Gandhi, Mussoorie Lecture, 29 May 1946 [117]

Gandhi, himself, never tried to convince others to be vegetarian.

> *Vegetarians need to be tolerant . . . adopt a little*
> *humility. We should appeal to the moral sense of*
> *the people who do not see eye to eye with us.*
>   Gandhi, *Harijan*,
>   20 February 1919 [118]

Gandhi felt that Hindus must never seek to convert others by force of arms, but rather by the wisdom of *ahimsa*.

> *They must rely upon the working of the great prin-*
> *ciple* [ahimsa] *in their own lives and making its*
> *effective appeal to the outer world. They will not*
> *convert the latter* [non-vegetarians] *by force of*
> *arms. They certainly can by the force of ahimsa.*
> *We little realize the matchless potency of ahimsa*
> *when it is thoroughly put into active operation.*
>   Gandhi, *Young India*,
>   11 November 1926 [119]

He believed, however, that, in the end

> [Hindus will guide] *the rest of the world to their*
> *way of thinking only by living the religion of*
> *ahimsa as fully as humanly possible.*
>   Gandhi, *Young India*,
>   11 November 1926 [120]

PART FOUR

SUMMARY &
CONCLUSION

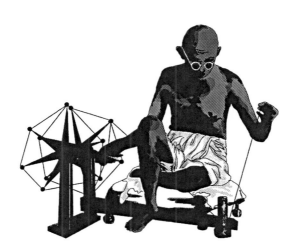

*The message of the spinning wheel is much
wider than its circumference. Its message is
one of simplicity, service of mankind, living
so as not to hurt others.*

Gandhi, *Young India,*
17 September 1925 [1]

SUMMARY & CONCLUSION

CHAPTER 9: MAHATMA GANDHI: THE VEGETARIAN

GANDHI'S MESSAGE OF NON-VIOLENCE, NON-ABUNDANCE & MERCIFUL LIVING

Mahatma Gandhi began his life, lived his life, and departed from this life as a vegetarian. As a young child, Gandhi observed, and then absorbed, the vegetarian values of his parents, family and community. The values that were shown him were Hindu values of non-violence, non-abundance and compassion for the soul of God within all beings.

Young Gandhi fully accepted the values of the vegetarian environment in which he had been raised. He recognized that these vegetarian values were not values motivated by a quest for personal health, but rather by selfless concerns for the welfare of other, more vulnerable beings. Gandhi so respected these values that he vowed to his mother never to consume the flesh of weaker beings.

Yet young Gandhi still wondered if his decision was one of free choice, or one that had been so instilled in him by his heritage that he could not recognize its underlying truths or untruths.

Then one day, while a student in London, he purchased a book for one shilling titled, *Salt's Plea for Vegetarianism*. He read the book from cover to cover. It solidified his conviction that it is morally incumbent upon vegetarians not to live upon the flesh of their fellow beings.

> *From the day of reading this book, I may claim to have become a vegetarian by choice.*
>
> Gandhi, *Key to Health* [2]

Although Gandhi blessed the day he vowed before his mother to remain vegetarian, it was not until that day that he finally made the conscious decision to remain vegetarian of his own free will, that it became a spiritual, moral commitment.

> *Choice was now made in favor of vegetarianism, the spread of which henceforth became my mission.*
>
> Gandhi, *Key to Health* [3]

Gandhi's personal choice to live as a vegetarian was related neither to issues of health nor of strength, but rather to an inner calling to protect the life of any and all weaker beings.

> *The basis of my vegetarianism is not physical, but moral. If anybody said that I should die if I did not take beef tea or mutton, even under medical advice, I would prefer death. That is the basis of my vegetarianism.*
>
> Gandhi, *Key to Health* [4]

Mahatma Gandhi's commitment to vegetarianism and non-violence towards all created beings became a lifelong passion.

> *At an early age, in the course of my experiments, I found that a selfish basis would not serve the purpose of taking a man higher and higher along the paths of evolution. What was required was an altruistic purpose.*
>
> Gandhi, *Harijan*, 20 February 1919 [5]

Gandhi's personal vegetarian philosophy evolved slowly. It grew as an amalgam of ideals, lessons, and spiritual awakenings. Gandhi felt the longing needs of the most vulnerable amongst society and the most loathed amongst creation. He harbored love, respect, and compassion for all.

> *I still continue to hold life not only in man and animal, but in plant and flower as sacred.*
>
> Gandhi, *Discourses on the Gita*, 28 November 1926 [6]

His vegetarian philosophy was an expression of the compassion he felt for all vulnerable and weaker beings

> *Taught by the Power that pities me, I learn to pity them.*
>
> Gandhi, Right to Live, *Harijan*, 9 January 1937 [7]

Gandhi encouraged people to rid themselves of any feelings of superiority, or any urge to dominate other beings. He guided people to show the same mercy towards all beings, that these same people begged God to show them.

Ahimsa is not a mere matter of dietetics, it transcends it. What a man eats or drinks matters little; it is the self-denial, the self-restraint behind it that matters. [A man's goal is] *Ahimsa . . . if his heart overflows with love and melts at another's woe.*

Gandhi, *Young India*, 6 September 1928 [8]

Although Gandhi was initially led to vegetarianism out of respect for his family, as his spiritual and moral philosophy matured, he remained committed to vegetarianism because of his strong beliefs in non-violence, his commitment to non-abundance, his wish not to possess that which others had no chance of ever possessing, his desire not to take more from creation than he absolutely needed, and his passion to live without taking the breath of life from any being. These were the vegetarian values that emerged, evolved, and filled his commitment with meaning.

Our dominion over the lower order of creation is not for their slaughter, but for their benefit equally with ours. For I am certain that they are endowed with a soul as I am.

Gandhi, *Young India*, 17 December 1925 [9]

CHAPTER 10: MAHATMA GANDHI: "THE GREAT SOUL"

The wisdom of Gandhi is both profound and practical. Although grounded in worldly truths, it contains an essence of other-world spirituality.

> *God is neither in heaven, nor down below, but in everyone.*
>
> Gandhi, *My God* [10]

Throughout his life, Gandhi sought to give hope to the people of India so they could cultivate the inner fortitude to fight for independence through non-violent means.

He sought to imbue them with a sense of shared commitment and concern for all people, all beings, and all creation.

Gandhi loved his people, his country, and even his enemy. He recognized that to love others, one must humble oneself below them.

> *A man who wants to love the whole world, including one who calls himself his enemy, knows how impossible it is to do so on his own strength. He must be as mere dust before he can understand the elements of Ahimsa. He is nothing if he does not daily grow in humility as he grows in love.*
>
> Gandhi, Plea for Humility,
> *Young India*, 25 June 1925 [11]

The core of Gandhi's philosophy, from which all the other philosophical concepts grew, was humbleness.

> *Bowing to the earth we learn to be humble even as the earth is humble. She supports the beings that tread upon her. We are of the earthly earth. If earth is not, we are not. I feel nearer God by feeling Him through the Earth. In bowing to the Earth, I at once realize my indebtedness to Him and if I am a worthy child of that Mother, I shall at once reduce myself to dust and rejoice in establishing kinship with the lowest forms of creation whose fate—reduction to dust—I have to share with them.*
>
> Gandhi, Bapu's Letters to Mira,
> 1 December 1931 [12]

Gandhi recognized that in his struggle to secure non-violent change, without the strength of humbleness, neither he nor his people would succeed.

> *If one has pride and egoism, there is no non-violence. Non-violence is impossible without humility.*
>
> Gandhi, *Harijan*, 28 January 1939 [13]

And if humankind does not recognize that it must coexist peacefully with the other beings with whom it shares this planet, it will destroy itself.

> *So long as a man does not of his own free will put himself last among his fellow creatures, there is no salvation for him.*
>
> Gandhi, *Autobiography* [14]

Gandhi felt a profound need to help the suffering masses of humanity, and not inflict any harm upon humankind's brethren beings within the vast animal kingdom.

His belief in the *Law of Karma* and the *Law of Rebirth* reinforced his conviction that all beings were created by God, all possessed the soul of God, and, all are of God. He felt that as God created all life, only God possessed the right to take such life.

He believed that in the ever-turning cycle of *karma* and rebirth, all people share responsibility for the fate of all others, and must feel that same compassion for all humanity and all creatures, as for themselves, as all are of the same essence.

> *Certainly, the lower creatures are as brethren to us. We all come from the same source.*
>
> Gandhi, *Discourses on the Gita*,
> 15 June 1926 [15]

Gandhi was saddened and humbled by the realization that to sustain his own existence, some *himsa* was inherently necessary.

> *I am painfully aware of the fact that my desire to continue life in the body involves me in constant himsa. . . . For instance, I know that in the act of respiration I destroy innumerable invisible germs floating in the air. But I do not stop breathing. The consumption of vegetables involves himsa, but I find that I cannot give them up. Again, there is himsa in the use of antiseptics, yet I cannot bring myself to discard the use of disinfectants like kerosene, etc., to rid myself of the mosquito pest and the like. . . Thus there is no end of himsa which I directly and indirectly commit.*
>
> Gandhi, *Young India,* 1 November 1928 [16]

Gandhi's belief in non-violence, *ahimsa,* became a personal creed. It included love, truth, service, consideration, non-hurtful deeds, sincere words, and tender tolerance for differences, as well as moderation in wants.

He considered not hurting any living being an essential component of his philosophy of *ahimsa.* He felt that the essence of *ahimsa* was assaulted by every evil thought, every thought of hatred, every ill wish against another, and every desire of hold to oneself that which the world needs.[17] Gandhi oftentimes spoke of *ahimsa* as the means and Truth as the end.[18]

> *In this world we cannot live without truth and nonviolence.*
>
> Gandhi, Prayer Meeting, New Delhi,
> 30 October 1947 [19]

Gandhi did not foresee in the near future a time when all the world, or for that matter, all of India, would follow *ahimsa*. Yet, he longed for a time when humankind would recognize the power of God within each individual, and hence, rely less upon physical force and more upon soul-force.[20] He advised people to recognize they were instruments of God and attempt to live following God's acts of kindness,

> *I verily believe that man's habit of killing man on the slightest pretext has darkened his reason and he gives himself liberties with other life which he would shudder to take if he really believed that God was a God of Love and Mercy.*
> Gandhi, *Harijan*, 9 January 1937 [21]

Gandhi believed that to follow a life path of non-violence, one must possess a strong faith in God. That is because God, rather than weapons or bombs, must be one's strength.

Thus it is, that Gandhi is remembered as a man of pure, unconditional love, non-violence, non-abundance, and compassion for all people, all beings, and all creation.

> *All I claim for myself is that I am ceaselessly trying to understand the implications of great ideals like ahimsa and to practice them in thought, word and deed. But I know that I have a long distance yet to cover in this direction.*
> Gandhi, *Young India,* 1 November 1928 [22]

On January 30, 1948, Gandhi met his death. He had just arrived at the prayer grounds. He placed his hands together. The sound of gunshot was heard. Gandhi was assassinated.

Gandhi died, however, as he had hoped, with the name of God, "*Hè Rama, Hè Rama*" [Oh God, Oh God] on his lips.[23]

During his lifetime, Gandhi succeeded in:

> Securing freedom for the people of India through non-violent means.
>
> Eliminating the stigma of untouchability.
>
> Spreading mutual tolerance between the various religious groups of India.
>
> And, in showing the world that peace can be obtained through non-violent means.

Let us hope that Gandhi's message of non-violence and compassion towards all beings, and its most tangible resultant effect, vegetarianism, will, someday, attain the same success.

Back Matter

Gandhi sought to live in non-abundance. He believed that every time one took more from the world than one needed, one inflicted unnecessary harm upon other people, other beings, and the planet .

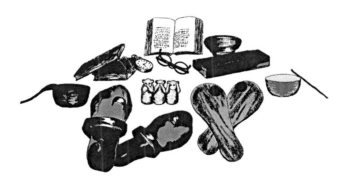

True to his word, when he died, Gandhi's only possessions were two pair of sandals, eating utensils, a watch, his eyeglasses, three holy books—the *Bhagavad Gita*, the *Bible*, and the *Koran*, and a small statue with three monkeys symbolizing, "See no evil, hear no evil, and speak no evil."

END NOTES

Unless stated otherwise, those articles, letters and speeches of Mahatma Gandhi not otherwise referenced, were retrived from the 100 volume compendium created by the Ministry of Information and Broadcasting of the Government of India, *The Collected Works of Mahatma Gandhi.*

INTRODUCTION
1 Gandhi, *Harijan*, 20 February 1919.
2 Gandhi, Mahatma, *The Bhagavad Gita According to Gandhi* (Edited by John Strohmeier. Berkeley, CA: Berkeley Hills Books, 2000), 234.
3 Gandhi, Letter to Avadhesh Dutt Avasthi, 24 May 1935.

PART ONE:
PLANTING OF SEEDS
1 Gandhi, *Harijan*, 20 February 1919.
2 Gandhi, Mahatma K. *Autobiography: The Story of My Experiments with Truth* (Translated by Mahadev Devi. NY: Dover Publications, 1983), 1–3.
3 Gandhi, *Autobiography*, 23.
4 Gandhi, *Prayer* (Compiled and edited by Chandrakant Kaji. Ahmedabad, India: Navajivan Publishing House, 1977. Reprint 1996), 171.
5 Gandhi, *Autobiography*, 55.
6 Gandhi, Speech at Islamia College, Peshawar, 1938.
7 Gandhi, *Key to Health* (Translated by Sushila Nayar. Ahmedabad, India: Navajivan Publishing House, 1948), 4.

8 Gandhi, *Autobiography*, 18.
9 Gandhi, *The Vegetarian*, 7 February 1891.
10 Gandhi, *Autobiography*, 208.
11 Gandhi, God Is, *Young India* 11 October 1928.
13 Gandhi, *Autobiography*, 105.
14 Richard Attenborough, T*he Words of Gandhi*, 2nd Ed. (NY: New market Press, 2000), 101.
15 Gandhi, *Young India*, 20 October 1927.
16 Gandhi, Discourses on the Gita, 4 July 1926.
17 Ibid.
18 Gandhi, *Young India*, 7 October 1926.
19 Gandhi, Speech at Tanjore, *Young India*, 29 September 1927.
20 Gandhi, *The Hindu*, 28 January 1933.
21 Gandhi, *Young India*, 7 October 1926.
22 Gandhi, *Harijan,* 26 December 1936.
23 Gandhi, Kottayam Speech, *Harijan*, 30 January 1937.
24 Gandhi, Speech at Public Meeting, Madras, *The Hindu*, 21 December 1933.

25 Gandhi, My Mission, *Young India*, 3 April 1924.

26 A. L. Basham, *The Wonder That was India*, 3rd Ed. (New Delhi: Rupa & Co., 2001. First published in 1954), 12.

27 Gandhi, *Harijan*, 30 January 1937.

28 Gandhi, *Epic of Travancore*, 174–180.

29 Gandhi, *Harijan*, 30 January 1937.

30 Gandhi, *Hindi Navajivan*, 31 October 1929.

31 Gandhi, More Animal that Human, *Young India*, 8 July 1926.

32 Gandhi, *Bhagavad Gita*, 17.

33 Swami Nikhilananda, *The Upanishads*, Vol I. (NY: Ramakrishna-Vivekananda Center, 1990), 32.

34 Gandhi, *Bhagavad Gita*, 150.

35 Gandhi, *Young India*, 21 October 1926.

36 Swami Sivananda, *All About Hinduism* (Tehri-Garhwal, U.P., Himalayas, India: Divine Life Society, 1997), 14.

37 Eknath Easwaran, *The Upanishads* (Tomales, CA: Nilgiri Press, 1987), 10–11.

38 Ibid., 36.

39 Gandhi, *Young India*, 5 June 1924

40 Sivananda, 75–82.

41 Gandhi, *Bhagavad Gita*, 89.

42 Gandhi, Letter to Devdas Gandhi, 24 July 1918.

43 Easwaran, *Upanishads*, 229.

44 Gandhi, *Bhagavad Gita*, 44.

45 Ibid., 102.

46 Sivananda, 66.

47 Gandhi, Diary of Mahadev Desai, 21 June 1932.

48 Gandhi, *Bhagavad Gita*, 234.

49 Gandhi, *Autobiography*, 20.

50 Gandhi, *Yeravda Mandir* (Ahmedabad, India: Navajivan Publishing House), 1935.

51 Gandhi, *Prayer*, 175–176.

52 Gandhi, *Young India*, 25 September 1925.

53 Gandhi, "Some Questions Answered," *Harijan*, 2 February 1934.

54 Gandhi, Letter to Raojibhai Patel, 7 March 1914.

55 Gandhi, *Autobiography*, 18.

56 Padmanabh S, Jaini, *The Jaina Path of Purification* (New Delhi: Motilal Banarsidass, 1979), 167–168.

57 Max F. Muller, ed. *The Sacred Books of the East*, vol. XXII, Part I *Jaina Sutras* (New Delhi: Motilal Banarsidass, 1964. First published Oxford University Press, 1884), 202.

58 Ibid, vol. XLV, Part II, 307.

59 Padmanabh, 66.

60 Gandhi, Notes, *Young India*, 22 May 1924.

61 Gandhi, Hinduism, *The Star*, 10 March 1905.

62 Edward A Conze, *A Short History of Buddhism* (London: George Allen & Unwin, 1980), 153.

63 Ainslie T Embree, *Sources of Indian Tradition*, 2nd Ed., Vol I. (NY: Columbia University Press, 1988. First Edition 1958), 170.

64 Conze, 153.

65 Wm. Theodore, De Bary ed. *Sources of Indian Tradition*, Vol. I (NY: Columbia University Press, 1985), 26.

66 De Bary, 169-170.

67 Basham, 282.

68 Gandhi, *Autobiography*, 140.

69 Gandhi, Speech at Young Men's Buddhist Association, Colombo, 25 November 1927.

70 Gandhi, Speech at Public Meeting, Badulla, 19 November 1927.

71 Seshagiri K. L. Rao, 2nd Ed. *Mahatma Gandhi and Comparative Religion* (New Delhi: Motilal Banarsidass Publishers, 1990), 151.

72 Rao, 31.

73 Gandhi, Speech at Public Meeting, Kottayam, *Harijan*, 30 January 1937.

74 Attenborough, 62.

75 *Open Bible*, King James Version, Publisher (Nashville, TN: Thomas Nelson Publishers, 1982), 1374.

76 Gandhi, Is Non-violence Effective? *Harijan*, 7 January 1939

PART TWO: CULTIVATION OF VALUES

1 Gandhi, Letter to the Viceroy, Lord Irwin, 2 March 1930.

2 Gandhi, *My God* (Ahmedabad, India: Navajivan Publishing House, 1962), 48.

3 Gandhi. Why I am a Hindu, *Young India*, 20 October 1927.

4 Gandhi, Speech at Aranmula, 20 January 1937.

5 Gandhi, *Autobiography*, 454.

6 *The Selected Works of Mahatma Gandhi*. Vol. Three. *Basic Works*. (General editor Shriman Narayan. Ahmedabad, India: Navajivan Publishing House, 1968), 221.

7 Gandhi, *Harijan*, 6 March 1939.

8 Gandhi, More Animal than Human, *Young India*, 8 July 1926.

9 Gandhi, Reason vs. Faith, *Young India*, 14 January 1927.

10 Gandhi, *A Thought for a Day*. Compiled by Anand T. Hingorani. (New Delhi: Ministry of Information & Broadcasting, Government of India, 1969), 427.

11 Gandhi, Ashram Observances in Action (1959).

12 Gandhi, Speech at Lausanne, 8 December 1931.

13 Gandhi, Discourses on the Gita, 28 November 1926

14 Gandhi, *Young India*, 4 October 1928

15 Gandhi, talk to Khudai Khidmagars, *Pilgrimage for Peace*, 87–91.

16 Gandhi, Sevagram, 5 August 1940.

17 Gandhi, Reply to Address at Bijapur, *The Hindu*, 3 June 1921.

18 Gandhi, *The Selected Works of Mahatma Gandhi*. Vol. IV *Selected Letters*. Shriman Narayan, Ed. (Ahmedabad, India: Navajivan Publishing House, 1968), 305.

19 Gandhi, *Bhagavad Gita*, 17–19.
20 Gandhi, God of Love, Not War, *Harijan*, 5 September 1936.
21 Gandhi, *Young India*, 4 October 1928.
22 Gandhi, Talk to Khudai Khimatgars, *A Pilgrimage for Peace*, 23 October 1938.
23 Ibid.
24 Gandhi, To Gandhi Seva Sangh, *Harijan*, 4 November 1939.
25 Gandhi, *Young India*, 3 April 1924.
26 Gandhi, Talk to Khudai Khimatgars, *A Pilgrimage for Peace*, 23 October 1938.
27 Gandhi, *Autobiography*, 454.
28 Gandhi, *Young India*, 3 September 1922.
29 Gandhi, Right to Live, *Harijan*, 9 January 1937.
30 Gandhi, *Young India*, 21 October 1926
31 Gandhi, *Young India*, 8 June 1921.
32 Gandhi, *Young India*, 16 June 1924.
33 Gandhi, *Young India*, 20 October 1927.
34 Gandhi, Save the Cow, *Young India*, 8 June 1921.
35 Gandhi, *Young India*, 6 October 1921.
36 Gandhi, God of Love, Not War, *Harijan*, 5 September 1936.
37 Ashram Vows 1930. From the weekly discourses at Yeravda Jail. *Hindu Dharma* (Ahmedabad, India: Navajivan Publishing House, 1950), 251.

38 Ibid, 254.
39 Gandhi, *Bhagavad Gita*, 20-23.
40 Ashram Vows 1930. From the weekly discourses at Yeravda Jail, 254.
41 Ibid, 255.
42 Gandhi, *My God*, 48.
43 Gandhi, *Young India*, 6 October 1921.
44 Gandhi, *Autobiography*, 235.
45 Gandhi, *Key to Health*, 13.
46 Gandhi, Letter to Maganlal Gandhi after 14 March 1915.
47 Catherine Clément, *Gandhi: Father of a Nation* (London: Thames and Hudson, 1996), 122.

PART THREE:
SPROUTING OF VALUES

1 Gandhi, *My Dear Child* (Ahmedbad, India: Navajivan Publishing House, 1956), 57
2 Gandhi, Letter to Ramdas Gandhi, 19 October 1934.
3 Gandhi, *Harijan*, 29 April 1933.
4 Gandhi, *Gandhi's Heath Guide*, 1.
5 Gandhi, *Young India*, 8 August 1929.
6 Ashram Vows 1930. From the weekly discourses at Yeravda Jail, 251.
7 Gandhi, *Harijan*, 7 April 1946.
8 Gandhi, *Key to Health*, 30.
9 Gandhi, *Young India*, 8 August 1929.

10 Gandhi, *Gandhi's Health Guide* (Freedon, CA: The Crossings Press, 2000), 2.

11 Gandhi, Talks to Ashram Women, 1926.

12 Gandhi, *Autobiography*, 287.

13 Gandhi, *Bhagavad Gita*, 137.

14 Ibid.

15 Gandhi, *Gandhi's Health Guide*, 188.

16 Gandhi, *Harijan*, 20 February 1919.

17 Ibid.

18 Gandhi, Letter to Aprakash Chandra Mehta, 2 August 1935.

19 Gandhi, Letter to S. Ambujammal, 5 May 1935.

20 Gandhi, Ashram Observances, *Character and Nation Building*. Edited by Valji Govindji Desai. (Ahmedabad, India: Navajivan Publishing House, 1959), 7.

21 Gandhi, *Key to Health*, 1.

22 Ibid., 1.

23 Ibid., 3.

24 Ibid., 3.

25 Ibid., 6.

26 Ibid., 7.

27 Gandhi, *Harijan*, 1 February 1935.

28 Gandhi, *Gandhi's Health Guide*, 111.

29 Gandhi, *Key to Health*, 10.

30 Ibid.

31 Gandhi, Letter to Ambujammal, 5 May 1935

32 Gandhi, *Harijan*, 25 January 1935.

33 Gandhi, *Key to Health*, 10.

34 Ibid., 11.

35 Gandhi, *Gandhi's Health Guide*, 79.

36 Ibid., 110–111.

37 Ibid., 97.

38 Ibid., 78.

39 Gandhi, *Harijan*, 19 October 1935.

40 Gandhi, *Young India*, 18 July 1929.

41 Ibid., 7 October 1926.

42 Ibid., 15 November 1928.

43 Gandhi, *Harijan*, 15 February 1935

44 Gandhi, *Key to Health*, 12.

45 Gandhi, *Young India*, 13 June 1929.

46 Gandhi, *Harijan*, 20 February 1919

47 Ibid.

48 Ibid.

49 Gandhi, *Gandhi's Health Guide*, 106.

50 Gandhi, *Young India*, 22 August 1929.

51 Gandhi, *Harijan*, 25 January 1942.

52 Gandhi, *Key to Health*, 12.

53 Ibid., 14.

54 Ibid., 12.

55 Gandhi, *Harijan*, 2 November 1935.

56 Ibid., 14 April 1946.

57 Gandhi, *Autobiography*, 239.

58 Gandhi, *Key to Health*, 8.

59 Gandhi, *Autobiography*, 59.

60 Gandhi, *Key to Health*, 7–8.

61 Ibid.

62 Gandhi, *Young India*, 18 July 1929.

63 Gandhi, *Key to Health*, 7–8.

64 Gandhi, *Harijan*, 13 October 1946.

65 Gandhi, Letter to D. B. Kalelkar and B. D. Kalelkar, 19 February 1933.

66 Gandhi, *Nature Cure*. Edited by Bharatan Kumarappa (Ahmedabad, India: Navajivan Publishing House, 1954), 56.

67 Gandhi, *Young India*, 22 August 1929.

68 Gandhi, Letter to Bal Kalelkar, 12 February 1933.

69 Ibid.

70 Gandhi, *Key to Health*, 13.

71 Gandhi, *Young India*, 18 July 1929.

72 Gandhi, *Key to Health*, 15.

73 Ibid.

74 Gandhi, *Key to Health*, 18 December 1942.

75 Ibid.

76 Gandhi, *Key to Health*, 17.

77 Ibid., 9 October 1942.

78 Ibid.

79 Ibid.

80 Gandhi, *The Moral Basis of Vegetarianism* (Ahmedabad, India: Navajivan Publishing House, 1959), 4.

81 Gandhi, *Young India*, 14 August 929.

82 Gandhi, *The Vegetarian Messenger*, 1 June 1891.

83 Gandhi, *The Vegetarian*, 21 February 1891.

84 Gandhi, *Gandhi's Health Guide*, 75.

85 Ibid., 77.

86 Ibid., 79.

87 Gandhi, *The Bhagavad Gita*, 208.

88 Gandhi, *Young India*, 15 August 1929.

89 Gandhi, *Autobiography*, 287.

90 Gandhi, *Young India*, 7 October 1926.

91 Ibid., 5 April 1926.

92 Gandhi, *Key to Health*, 8.

93 Gandhi, *The Bhagavad Gita*, 63.

94 Gandhi, *Key to Health*, 14.

95 Ibid., 13.

96 Gandhi, *Young India*, 8 August 1929.

97 Gandhi, Discourses on the Gita, 4 July 1926.

98 Gandhi, *Key to Health,* 14.

99 Gandhi, *Autobiography*, 240.

100 Gandhi, *Harijan*, 20 February 1919.

101 Ibid.

102 Gandhi, Letter to Jamnadas Gandhi, 17 March 1914.

103 Gandhi, *Harijan*, 2 February 1935.

104 Gandhi, *Key to Health*, 134 .

105 Ibid., 13.

106 Gandhi, *Autobiography*, 294.

107 Ibid., 287.

108 Gandhi, *Key to Health*, 14.

109 Gandhi, *Autobiography*, 292.

110 Gandhi, *Young India*, 24 March 1920.

111 Gandhi, *Autobiography*, 296.

112 Ibid., 297.

113 Ibid., 286.

114 Gandhi, *Discourses on the Gita*, 4 February 1926.

115 Gandhi, *Harijan*, 20 February 1919.

116 Gandhi, *Young India*, 23 September 1926.

117 Gandhi, Mussoorie Lecture, 29 May 1946.

[118] Gandhi, *Harijan*,
20 February 1919.
[119] Gandhi, *Young India,*
11 November 1926.
[120] Ibid.

PART FOUR:
SUMMARY & CONCLUSION

[1] Gandhi, *Young India*,
17 September 1925.
[2] Gandhi, *Key to Health*, 6.
[3] Ibid., 6.
[4] Ibid., 11.
[5] Gandhi, *Harijan*,
20 February 1919.
[6] Gandhi, *Discourses on the Gita*,
28 November 1926.
[7] Gandhi, Right to Live, *Harijan*,
9 January 1937.
[8] Gandhi, *Young India*,
6 September 1928.
[9] Ibid., 17 December 1925.
[10] Gandhi, *My God*, 48.

[11] Gandhi, Plea for Humility, *Young India*, 25 June 1925.
[12] Gandhi, Bapu's Letters to Mira,
1 December 1931.
[13] Gandhi, *Harijan*, 28 January 1939.
[14] Gandhi, *Autobiography*, 454.
[15] Gandhi, Discourses on the Gita,
15 June 1926.
[16] Gandhi, *Young India*,
1 November 1928.
[17] Gandhi, *Character and Nation Building*, 4–5.
[18] Gandhi, *Truth is God*, 35.
[19] Gandhi, Prayer Meeting,
New Delhi, 30 October 1947.
[20] Fischer, Louis. *Gandhi: His Life and Message for the World* (NY: New American Library, 1954), 131.
[21] Gandhi, *Harijan*, 9 January 1937.
[22] Gandhi, *Young India*,
1 November 1928.
[23] Clément, 113.
[24] [Closing page] Gandhi, *Harijan*,
24 March 1946.

GLOSSARY OF TERMS

Ahimsa: Non-violence in thought, word and deed.

Aryans: Those people of ancient times native to Northwest India who transmitted the wisdom of the *Vedas*.

Ayurvedic Medicine: An ancient system of traditional Indian health care. *Ayus* means life and *veda* means knowledge. Ayurvedic medicine incorporates healthy living, massage, herbs, and oils to keep the body in physical, mental, and spiritual harmony.

Asafetida: A bitter resinous roots of several plants in the parsley family.

Bajri: A type of flour popular in the villages of India.

Bhagavad Gita: One of the great Hindu epics derived from another larger epic, the *Mahabharata*. It teaches the values of renunciation, the *Laws of Karma* and *Rebirth*, and of the tragedies of war and violence.

Buddha (Gautama Siddhartha): Founder of the Buddhist faith. Gautama Buddha was born in 563 BCE in Southern Nepal, the son of a Hindu chieftain.

Buddhism: The philosophy of morality, *karma*, and cyclic rebirth formulated by Gautama Buddha during the sixth to fifth century BCE.

Caste System: An ancient Indian system from Vedic times classifying society into four main groups: *brahmin, kshatriya, vaishya*, and *shudra* (untouchables).

Dharma: One's spiritual duty. The responsibility one has to fulfill one's destiny.

Epicarp: The outermost layer of the pericarp of a fruit.

Gur: Unrefined whole sugar.

Haricot Bean: A variety of green bean that is longer and thinner than traditional green beans.

Himsa: Any act of violence including violent thoughts, words, and actions.

Indus Valley Civilization: The ancient Indian civilization of the Indus River Valley in Northwest India.

Jain Faith: One of India's most ancient traditions. It is a nontheistic faith that places great emphasis upon concepts of *karma*, rebirth and nonviolence towards all beings.

Jambu: A white to light red fruit with a thin, shiny shell.

Karma: A foundational Hindu belief that one's actions in prior lives affect one's fate in one's present and future lives. The term *karma* refers both to one's actions and to the results of one's actions.

Mahabharata: One of the great Indian epics (the *Ramayana,* and *Bhagavad Gita* being the others), tracing spiritual and karmic events amongst a group of family members. Its teachings have contributed to the formation of Hindu philosophy.

Mahavira: Born 468 BCE. Most recent spiritual guide of the Jain faith.

Masoor: A greenish-brown bean similar to lentils.

Moosambi: A citrus fruit, also termed "sweet lime."

Pericarp: The tissue surrounding a seed. In fleshy fruits, the pericarp contains three layers. Epicarp is the outer tough layer. The mesocarp is the middle fleshy layer forming the fruit. The endocarp is the inner membranous layer surrounding the seed.

Pulse: The edible seed of certain pod-bearing plants, such as peas or beans.

Puranas: A voluminous source of Hindu doctrine and mythology containing philosophical and spiritual teachings that have guided Hindu thought for generations.

Ramayana: One of India's great epics (the *Mahabharata* and *Bhagavad Gita* being the others). It traces the fate of the soul (represented by *Sita*) and has contributed to the formation of present day Hindu philosophical thought.

Rishi: Those individuals of ancient times considered seers of truth through whom God transmitted the *Vedas*, to share this wisdom with humankind.

Swaraj: Freedom from oppression by others.

Upanishads: The final portion of each of the *Vedas*. The *Upanishads* contain the essence of Hinduism's philosophical and metaphysical principles.

Vedas: The most ancient of all Hindu writings. They are perceived as containing wisdom revealed by God. The four *Vedas* are the *Rg Veda, Yajur Veda, Sama Veda, Artharva Veda*.

Vaishnava Hindu Faith: One of the principal traditions of Hinduism. Vishnu is worshiped as the supreme God. Vaishnava theology includes concepts of *karma*, reincarnation, and several systems of yoga.

REFERENCES

EXPLANATION OF COMMON REFERENCE SOURCES

*Collected Works of Mahatma Gandh*i

The official compendium of Gandhi's articles, letter,
and speeches retrived to date.
Created by the Ministry of Information and Broadcasting
of the Government of India

The *Collected Works of Mahatma Gandh*i is the official compendium containing all the speeches ever voiced and all the articles and letters ever written by Mahatma Gandhi, retrieved to date. Its creation has been a dedicated project by the Government of India since Mahatma Gandhi's death. The articles within the *Collected Works* are arranged chronologically according to when they were created.

The *Collected Works* presently consists of one hundred volumes of approximately 500 pages each. It was begun under a directive from the then Prime Minister of India, Jawaharlal Nehru, to ensure that all of Gandhi's writings and speeches would be retained throughout posterity. Many are articles that Gandhi wrote for periodicals, including *Harijan* and *Young India.*

Quotations from the *Collected Works* cited within this book are referenced according to the date they were created. They are not referenced according to the specific volume and page in which they appear, because these are continually changing, and will continue to do so, as earlier writings are found and inserted in their correct chronological position within newer edition of the *Collected Works.*

REFERENCES

Attenborough, Richard. T*he Words of Gandhi*, 2nd Ed. NY: New-market Press, 2000.

Basham, A. L. *The Wonder That was India*, 3rd Ed. New Delhi: Rupa & Co., 2001. First published in 1954.

Clément, Catherine. *Gandhi: Father of a Nation*. London: Thames and Hudson, Ltd., 1996.

Collected Works of Mahatma Gandhi. New Delhi: Publications Division, Ministry of Information & Broadcasting, Government of India. Second Revised Edition, 2000.

Conze, Edward. *A Short History of Buddhism*. London: George Allen & Unwin, 1980.

De Bary, Wm. Theodore, ed. *Sources of Indian Tradition*, Vol. I. NY: Columbia University Press, 1985.

Easwaran, Eknath. *The Upanishads*. Tomales, CA: Nilgiri Press, 1987.

Embree, Ainslie T. *Sources of Indian Tradition*, 2nd Ed., Vol I. NY: Columbia University Press, 1988. First Edition 1958.

Fischer, Louis. *Gandhi: His Life and Message for the World*. NY: New American Library, 1954.

Gandhi, Mahatma K. *Autobiography: The Story of My Experiments with Truth.* Translated by Mahadev Devi. NY: Dover Publications, 1983.

————. *The Bhagavad Gita According to Gandhi*. Edited by John Strohmeier. Berkeley, CA: Berkeley Hills Books, 2000.

———. *Character and Nation Building*. Edited by Valji Govindji Desai. Ahmedabad, India: Navajivan Publishing House, 1959.

———. *From Yeravda Mandir*, 2nd Ed. Ahmedabad, India: Navajivan Publishing House, 1935.

———. *Gandhi's Health Guide*, Freedon, CA: The Crossings Press, 2000.

———. *Hindu Dharma*. Ahmedabad, India: Navajivan Publishing House, 1950.

———. *Key to Health*. Translated by Sushila Nayar. Ahmedabad, India: Navajivan Publishing House, 1948.

———. *The Moral Basis of Vegetarianism*, Ahmedabad, India: Navajivan Publishing House, 1959.

———. *My Dear Child*. Ahmedabad, India: Navajivan Publishing House, 1956.

———. *My God*. Ahmedabad, India: Navajivan Publishing House, 1962.

———. *Nature Cure*. Edited by Bharatan Kumarappa. Ahmedabad, India: Navajivan Publishing House, 1954.

———. *Prayer*. Compiled and edited by Chandrakant Kaji. Ahmedabad, India: Navajivan Publishing House, 1977. Reprint 1996.

———. *The Selected Works of Mahatma Gandhi*. Volume Three. *The Basic Works*. General editor Shriman Narayan. Ahmedabad, India: Navajivan Publishing House, 1968.

———. *The Selected Works of Mahatma Gandhi*. Volume Four. *Selected Letters*. General editor Shriman Narayan. Ahmedabad, India: Navajivan Publishing House, 1968.

———. *A Thought for a Day*. Compiled by Anand T. Hingorani. New Delhi: Publications Division, Ministry of Information and Broadcasting, Government of India, 1969.

———. *Yeravda Mandir*. Ahmedabad, India: Navajivan Publishing House, 1935.

Harijan. A weekly journal edited by Mahatma Gandhi and others. Published in Ahmedabad, India. Unless otherwise specified, articles are located in the *Collected Works of Mahatma Gandhi*.

Jaini, Padmanabh S, *The Jaina Path of Purification*. New Delhi: Motilal Banarsidass, 1979.

Muller, Max F, ed. *The Sacred Books of the East*, Vol XXII, Part I. *Jaina Sutras*. New Delhi: Motilal Banarsidass, 1964. First published by Oxford University Press, 1884.

Muller, Max F, ed. *Sacred Books of the East, Jaina Sutras*. Vol XLV, Part II. New Delhi: Motilal Banarsidass, 1964. First published by Oxford University Press, 1895.

Nikhilananda, Swami. *The Upanishads*, Vol I. NY: Ramakrishna-Vivekananda Center, 1990.

Open Bible, King James Version, Publisher. Nashville, Tennessee: Thomas Nelson Publishers, 1982.

Rao, Seshagiri K.L., 2nd Ed. *Mahatma Gandhi and Comparative Religion*. New Delhi: Motilal Banarsidass Publishers, 1990.

Sivananda, Swami. *All About Hinduism*. Tehri-Garhwal, U.P., Himalayas, India: Divine Life Society, 1997.

Young India. Weekly journal edited by Mahatma Gandhi. Published in Ahmedabad, India. Unless otherwise specified, articles are located in the *Collected Works of Mahatma Gandhi*.

Ahimsa is the highest duty. Even if we cannot practice it in full, we must try to understand its spirit and refrain as far as is humanly possible from violence.

Gandhi, *Harijan*, 24 March 1946 [24]

Printed in the United States
86737LV00003B/256-312/A